# ANCIENT
# KNOWLEDGE

Distributed by
P & R Medical Services, Inc.
P.O. Box 262488
Plano, TX  75026
www.AncientTravels.com

This book is a work of fiction.  It is not intended for use in the actual treatment of patients.  Any similarity between the book's characters or events with real people or events is purely coincidental.

ISBN-13: 978-1466357853
ISBN-10: 1466357851

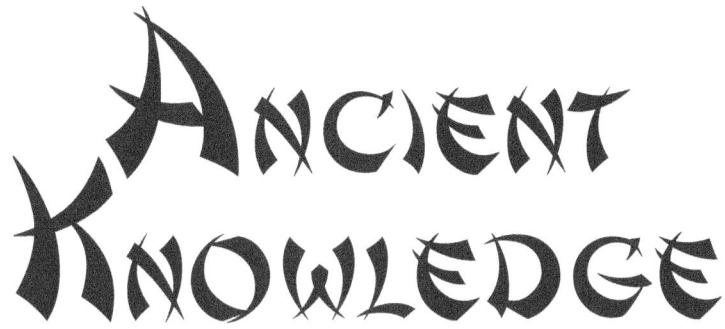

# Ancient Knowledge

Continuation of a Discourse Between a
Master and His Student on Acupuncture and
Chinese Martial Arts.

Richard A. Peck, L.Ac.

With Illustrations by Iva Lim Peck, L.Ac.

# EXCERPTS

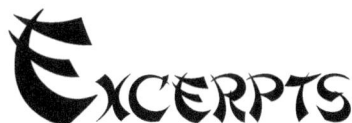

...It was unusual for him to feel this apprehension. His training in both external and internal Chinese martial arts prepared him for almost any situation, but as this shadow approached, the apprehension worsened.

...Some doctors try to treat all headaches or migraines the same way. In ancient China, however, doctors identified as many as twenty-one different reasons for a person to have this particular condition.

...There are usually two possible reasons for a sore throat, either an excess or a deficiency. In your case I suspect you have an excess of heat.

...Liu asked the young woman a series of questions similar to those he would ask of any woman he was examining. In addition, he asked her specific questions pertaining to her poor lactation.

...Liu sensed a change in the Universal Energy as they passed the portal.

...Painful Bi Syndrome is characterized by the patient complaining of severe stabbing pain in one or more joint.

...There are certain acupuncture points and Ahsi Points that are effective in self defense. I will teach you about them.

# PREFACE

avorable comments about my first book *Ancient Travels* encouraged me to write this sequel. Readers felt that blending martial arts and Traditional Chinese Medicine into the framework of a teaching novel was unique, interesting, and educational. As I look back on the start of the first novel, this has proved to be an effective way to convey my original intent which was to first teach and second to be entertaining.

Hopefully, with this book, *Ancient Knowledge*, readers will receive an even deeper understanding and appreciation of Traditional Chinese Medicine, Chinese martial arts, and the history and culture of China.

Those who read *Ancient Travels*, were also kind enough to give constructive suggestions for this sequel. Many suggested more martial arts, others were happy with the Chinese martial arts, but wanted additional and expanded concepts of Traditional Chinese Medicine. These comments and other suggestions were taken into consideration in the planning and writing of this book.

There are references made in this book to topics explained within the first book that the reader may want to explore further. To avoid boring the reader, I don't always revisit the information, but will occasionally make reference to the fact that the information has been related before. If the reader wants to know more about a particular topic then I strongly suggest reading the first book.

The main characters, Liu Bin and his young protégé Pei Ke, once again carry the story forward as they continue their travels. This time they are traveling from Liu's ancestral home to Beijing. As in the first book they are beset upon by those who want them killed.

I want to thank my wife, Iva Lim Peck, for allowing me to once again use one of her landscape paintings as a cover. I have also included some of her other paintings within the novel. As mentioned previously, I am indebted to my acupuncture and martial arts teachers for being so generous in sharing with me their knowledge and expertise. They imparted information that they rarely shared with others. To this day, I am amazed as to why they chose to share this Ancient Knowledge with me and not others. Hopefully, my writings and teachings will continue the process they started so many years ago.

I also want to thank Mat Rayback who helped me to impart the message I wanted to convey. It is interesting to see the final version once his editorial corrections are made. It is remarkably different than the initial draft. Mat has a wonderful way of taking thought patterns and blending them into a cohesive story.

I want to also thank my wife for making sure the concepts of Traditional Chinese Medicine, as explained within the story, are correct. I would also like to thank Victor Yannacone and his wife Carol for their reading of the book. From their first hand experience of Traditional Chinese Medicine, they have a wonderful insight into what is important to the reader and what is not important. I value their comments and have incorporated many of their suggestions into this book.

I want to thank Landa Miller who once again was kind enough to read the manuscript and make important recommendations. Her contribution to the book includes the back cover. Also, Jerry Robinson and David Pinkard were kind enough to help proof read the manuscript and make suggestions that enhanced the readability of the story.

Again, I want to thank the students and patients I have had over the years who unknowingly taught me so much about how to be a good practitioner of TCM and a teacher.

As I mentioned in the first book, this is strictly a work of fiction. There is no similarity between the characters mentioned in this book and any individuals past or present.

I have tried to accurately describe both the geographic locations in China and the concepts of Traditional Chinese Medicine. Any errors or omissions in this work are strictly of my own doing. Hopefully, you will enjoy this book like you did the first. I do value your comments.

Richard A. Peck, L.Ac. (February 2013)
www.AncientTravels.com
www.IntegratedCenterForOrientalMedicine.com

# PROLOGUE

Master Liu Bin and his protégé Pei Ke previously traveled north from the temple where he had lived for many years to Liu's ancestral village and home. His summons home came under unusual and peculiar circumstances. The note he received from an anonymous traveler was supposedly from his older brother. He had not seen his brother or his immediate family in years, but he would always recognize his brother's handwriting. What he looked at was not written by his brother.

In addition to the discrepancy in the writing, the tone of the note was quite disconcerting, suggesting he needed to return home as soon as possible. He realized after reading it that there was a shift in the Universal Energy. He had experienced these shifts, and knew from his past experience with Qi Gong and meditation that each shift was a response to something that had already happened or a precursor to something that was about to happen.

It was easy for Pei Ke to decide to follow Liu since his parents were deceased and his sister was happily married. There was no one else to keep him where he was except for the continued teachings of Liu. If he didn't follow Liu then, there would be nothing for him in that area.

As a dutiful student, he carried not only his own belongings but also those of his teacher, including an amulet. Unbeknown to him, the amulet was the potential key to the Liu family's vast fortune. He was charged with the responsibility of guarding the amulet and Liu's belongings at all times.

On the journey north, they were set upon in a series of attacks. Liu surmised the attacks had something to do with his return home. He didn't know why he was being attacked nor did he know by whom. Throughout the journey, Liu continued to teach Pei Ke the fundamentals of Traditional Chinese Medicine and the internal Chinese martial arts of Tai Chi Chuan, Pa Kua Chang, and Hsing-Yi Chuan.

Pei Ke's training had started two years previously, but was now being accelerated. Each day Liu introduced additional concepts of martial arts and Traditional Chinese Medicine. Thus Pei Ke's understanding of Yin Yang Theory, Five Element Theory, I Ching, Feng Shui, and other esoteric concepts were further enriched.

The more intensified and in-depth martial arts training made Pei Ke even more committed, and he rededicated himself to being a great martial artist and healer like his teacher.

Liu had made this trip before and knew the landmarks and places to stay where food and lodging were readily available. Invariably, at the end of each day, wherever they rested for the night, Liu found an opportunity to help others with their health care issues. This was part of the training Pei Ke received over the course of two or three weeks.

At one of their stops, they stayed with Liu's former student, now one of Liu's inner door students. There, Pei Ke met the daughter, Mei Li, and became smitten with her beauty and demeanor.

When they finally arrived at their destination, Liu learned from a trusted family friend, Mr. Wu, that most of his family, with the exception of one niece—Hua Yee—and a few younger children, were killed by assailants claiming ownership of the Liu family fortune and estate.

Although Pei Ke found Liu's niece attractive, protocol and the circumstances prevented him from pursuing a relationship.

During Liu's visit to his ancestral home, he found the fresh graves of his older brother and extended family. He paid his respects and vowed revenge. Their deaths seemed senseless to him.

Liu and Pei Ke followed the trail of Chen Su to avenge the death of his family. Pei Ke unintentionally helped with the process of avenging the deaths of Liu's family by killing one of the assailants. They returned to see Wu and Liu's niece, Hua Yee. She learned that Pei Ke who was a complete stranger to her had helped defend the family honor. She was immediately attracted to Pei Ke. Pei Ke in turn came to know Hua Yee better and became further attracted to her beauty and poise.

Liu settled the estate and made arrangements for Hua Yee and the other surviving family members. He left for unknown places with Pei Ke wondering what to do next. Part of him wanted to follow wherever Liu went and another part of him wanted to visit with Mei Li or Hua Yee. There were too many possibilities for him, and he was torn between them.

Liu knew Pei Ke had to make a decision whether to continue his studies or to pursue other interests. To further complicate Pei Ke's decision, Liu had offered Pei Ke the opportunity to inherit a vast fortune from the Liu estate. At Liu's request, Pei Ke visited the Abbot of the local temple, who helped him calm his anxiety and concerns about his teacher's whereabouts. Pei Ke awoke from a restful sleep knowing exactly what he needed to do next.

The story continues....

# CHAPTER ONE

As Liu Bin walked along the road to Beijing he sensed a profound shift in the Universal Energy. He had felt this shift before, but this time the shift was stronger than what he had ever experienced. Even though he could not immediately see them he instantly knew that those ominous and piercing eyes that had haunted him since leaving the temple for his ancestral home weeks before had something to do with the energy shift. They were once again looking at him from afar.

He sighed, but made no other sign that he knew the sinister and evil eyes were there. He shifted the sack on his back and continued walking deliberately and confidently down the curved and sloping road.

The road had split at the top of the hill, but he didn't hesitate in taking the left branch. From his previous experience traveling this road he knew it was more difficult and longer, but it was also more peaceful and more scenic.

In one of his previous journeys to Beijing he had taken the road to the right, but found it crowded with other travelers. He wanted peace and quiet from the interactions of the world. He wanted to enjoy the beauty of nature and would only get to assimilate this with the path he had chosen.

He almost always sought out the peaceful path in whatever he did. Many times the more peaceful endeavors in life were initially the most difficult. Such mutual qualities were in keeping with what he felt was the combination of Taoism, Buddhism, and the other philosophies he followed that fostered growth in the Universal Energy.

Thus the choice of using the road to the left was in actuality no choice at all. From years of experience he knew that the Universal Energy guided him on his course of action. He went with the flow of this powerful energy.

It was obvious those eyes knew exactly where he was going, though he couldn't guess how. He had shared his plans with no one except the Abbot of the temple and Mr. Wu, yet the sinister eyes seemed to know exactly what he was doing and where he was going.

Who were they, he wondered? What did they want? He began to feel uneasy. He knew events of the previous two months were not quite finalized, but he had thought that once he had accomplished his duty to his family, the eyes which came and went unexpectedly would be gone forever.

He was obviously wrong. He wondered if these eyes had anything to do with the discrepancy between what Hua Yee heard in the hiding place and what Wu told him he found when he examined the place. He had made note of the fact that Hua Yee mentioned there were three men looking for her. She could tell there were three by the differences in their voices. However, Mr. Wu only found two dead men at the scene. Either Hua Yee was mistaken on what she had heard or there were really three men at that time and one was now missing.

Maybe the eyes had something to do with Chen Su's son who had escaped the fight on the mountain? He had no idea where Chen Su's son was, but he was certain if he was still alive, sometime in the not too distant future they would meet. He realized that once they crossed paths there could be only one outcome. He didn't dwell on it often, but it was always in the back of his mind.

These were possibilities he knew he had to consider, but the energy he now sensed was different from what he had experienced in the last two months. The energy that had led to the challenge to the Liu ancestral lands and the cruel death of his brothers and their families had made a mark on his inner spirit. It had been evil and sinister, brought on by misguided hate and revenge. But he had dealt with it. He emerged victorious, not only for himself but for those remaining alive within the Liu legacy.

This new energy was clearly evil as well, out of harmony with the Yin Yang continuum, but it did not seem as sinister as the other. It was more cunning, more deceitful.

Liu stopped abruptly and quickly turned his head to the left. A movement in the forest had caught his eye. As quickly as it had come it disappeared behind a tree. A fraction of a second later the shape reappeared briefly, one tree closer. Liu's heart quickened as he sensed a greater unsettling in the overall Universal Energy.

It was unusual for him to feel this apprehension. His training in both external and internal Chinese martial arts prepared him for almost any situation, but as this shadow approached, the apprehension worsened. He could not quite make out the shape. It looked like a person, but the way it moved from one tree to another was not normal. There was a fluidity and stealth not usually seen in humans.

His pulse quickened and he felt chills run down his spine as a deep coldness descended on him. He watched with growing alarm as the shape progressed from one tree to another, getting ever so close. Liu had never run from an altercation, but this moving shape was unnatural.

He remembered the stories he had heard and the books he had read about people on the dark side. He'd never paid them much heed, considering them tales from people with overzealous imaginations. Now he wondered if this shape and its eerie movements were part of the dark side. If it was, then he would need to draw on all his abilities to defeat it.

As the shape moved from one tree to another, Liu also heard a rustling of leaves behind him and the sound of fast approaching footsteps. As they drew closer, he raised both arms in the preparatory Dragon Palm position of Pa Kua Chang. He turned and rooted his body to the Yin energy of the earth as he faced what he was sure was an attack.

For a fraction of a second, he forgot the eyes and the shape in the forest closing in on him. He needed to concentrate on this new threat. His attacker was young, but moved like a well-conditioned martial artist.

Liu moved quickly to keep his opponent from fixing a linear attack on him. Liu knew from years of practice and experience in similar situations that his opponent had to continually adjust the angle of attack to compensate for Liu's changing position. As long as Liu kept moving he had an advantage.

The lunge was unexpected. The attacker charged toward Liu with his head bowed slightly forward. Liu had expected a punch or a kick. He chastised himself for not being prepared for this. It was obvious that the attacker's goal was to take him down to the ground, but wrestling was the last thing Liu wanted to do. Once on the ground, he would be at the mercy of not only the attacker but also of any other attackers who might be waiting for an advantage. The eyes were still out there after all, and he didn't know if they had come any closer.

Liu stepped slightly to the right as he felt the arms of the attacker starting to encircle him. He rooted his weight on his back foot and used a variation of the Hsing-Yi Chuan move Bung Chuan to block downward and sideways against the attacker's head. Liu made sure that even though it was a downward block there was a rotation to his forearm as he made contact with the assailant. The force of the blow caught the opponent off guard. His forward momentum was diverted leftward causing him to fall forward and to the side of Liu.

Liu lifted his right hand and formed an eagle beak. His father had taught him how to put his fingers and thumb together in such a way that it resembled the beak of an eagle. Liu remembered how the eagle attacks and a fight could be stopped with one blow to one or more specific points on the body, and he now used this technique on the attacker.

Liu chose his point carefully. When the blow made contact with the soft tissue, Liu felt the energy shift in his opponent. His father's technique had been handed down within the family for generations. Liu remembered the day that his father showed him how to use the technique and the possible repercussions. The technique allowed him to kill, permanently paralyze his opponent, or simply knock him unconscious. Liu held all life sacred, so his strike merely stunned the man. He would soon regret his decision.

He heard movement off to the left somewhere in the trees. He turned quickly but could see nothing, not even the shape he saw before. He knew his position on the road was tenuous. He could stay and fight this evil or he could move on and face it another time.

Regaining his calm, he moved quickly down the road looking back occasionally to make sure he wasn't being followed. After ten minutes, he stepped off the road and concealed himself in the forest, to be certain he was not being followed.

He waited for what appeared to be an extended period of time, but no one came, so cautiously he went back to the road and looked back the way he'd come. He was uneasy. The Universal Energy had not yet righted itself, but he saw no one, so he continued warily on his journey.

As he had feared, no sooner was he back on the road than he was attacked again. It was the same attacker, but this time he wasn't alone. A second man charged beside him. Liu did not see where they'd emerged from, but it didn't matter now. He was not surprised and as he turned to meet them, he decided to stop these attacks for good. He no longer would be passive in his response to those that wanted to do harm to him and his family. This was his turning point. He had had enough of the evil energy and the attackers he assumed were associated with the energy. He would make peace with the Universal Energy later.

The first attacker, the one Liu had stunned, punched at Liu's face as the second grabbed his right arm. Liu dodged the punch, knocking it aside with a quick movement of his left hand.

The newcomer who'd grabbed Liu's arm was grinning wildly at his perceived advantage, completely oblivious of the death he'd brought on himself. With a quick Chin Na movement, Liu locked out the man's arm, exposing his head. Liu punched him quickly on the temple, close to the beginning of one of the classical meridians in Traditional Chinese Medicine. The man gasped and collapsed, dead.

Liu knew many of these points, but this one was fast and easy to execute. And it put him in the perfect position to deal with the other man.

He knew a stationary position was difficult to defend. He needed to keep moving, so he stepped sideways, dodging a snap kick to the groin. He timed the move perfectly to allow him to grab the opponent's extended foot. Many fighters would simply block such an attack, but Liu had learned to redirect the force of the kick with his arm making sure that it was a redirect and not a forceful block. This concept of redirect was more than just a deflection. It was a process of taking the opponents linear energy and diffusing it with circular energy.

With the energy dissipated Liu stepped slightly forward to quickly close the distance. With one foot he swept the man off his feet. With his free hand he grabbed the man's shirt and threw him forcefully to the ground.

Normally, this wouldn't have been fatal except Liu positioned his knuckles in such a way that when the man hit the ground Liu drove the concentrated force deep into a specific acupuncture point on the man's chest. Liu knew it would be fatal.

As his fist crushed into the acupuncture point, Liu heard the air being expelled from the man's chest. The man's eyes widened with fear. The pain spread in a direct line from the acupuncture point on the front of his body through his body to his spine. A combination of pain and energy exploded upwards to his head and downwards to his tail bone. Very few had ever felt the concentrated power of a Hsing-Yi Chuan punch, given at maximum intent, and lived to tell about it. This man would be no exception.

"Who sent you?" hissed Liu. "Tell me now or you will die." Liu already knew the man was dying when he raised his right hand high into the air, ready to strike the man.

The man gasped repeatedly for air as blood trickled from the side of his mouth and slowly rolled down his cheek. He looked frantically at Liu's fist and he began to whisper and gasp. Liu knew he didn't have much time before the man was dead.

"Who sent you?" Liu said again, threatening once more to hit the man.

The man gasped something, but it was barely audible through the gurgling sounds. Liu put his ear closer to the man's face to hear. He smelled of mud, sweat, and blood.

"Chen Chang," the man whispered.

"Who is Chen Chang?"

"The son of Chen Su," the attacker said. "He wants revenge for the killing of his father. He knows where you are going. He's put out a reward for you and your student. He wants you killed. You'll never make it to your destination alive. There are too many of us, waiting for you along the road."

Liu momentarily sat back. This was hardly a surprise. He'd known that someday he would again have to visit with the evilness of Chen Su. He knew he'd killed Chen Su, but the son had escaped. There was nothing he could have done about it at the time. He had hoped the winter weather would have caught the man unprepared and that he had died from exposure. He turned back to the dying man on the road and leaned close again.

"Where is Chen Chang now?" he asked.

"Following you to Bei…" The words became slurred and inaudible and with a final gurgle and gasp of air, he twitched and succumbed to the fatal blow. Liu felt the man's wrist for a pulse, but there was none to feel. He moved his hand to the attacker's face and closed the man's eyes. There was a slight positive change in the Universal Energy as the dead man's spirit rose from the road and departed to become part of another energy cycle. Liu leaned back on his heels, looking up and down the road.

So Chen Su's son's name was Chen Chang and he was still alive and was bent on revenge. Or, Liu mused, he might still believe that he had a rightful claim to Liu's ancestral lands. Liu thought for a moment.

If Chen Chang knew where he was going, the information had to have come from someone at the temple. Or the information came from Wu. He quickly dismissed the latter, as Wu would never tell anyone where he was going. He also dismissed the idea the Abbot told someone. He would have no reason to tell anyone. It was a mystery like the mystery that had originally summoned him home. He took a deep breath and stood up. He looked to the forest but saw nothing.

"I will be patient," he said aloud. "A solution will present itself."

The decision now was whether to return to his village to protect his student and the others, or continue on his travels to Beijing. His attacker had mentioned Pei Ke in the reward.

He looked at the bodies on the road. It was truly a waste that they died. They didn't even know why they died. Liu decided to leave the bodies where they fell. Maybe if they were found by Chen Chang's followers, it would give them second thought as to whether or not they really want to pursue him.

He turned and looked once again into the forest but could not see or sense anything out of the ordinary. With one final glance back down the road, he turned and continued on his way toward Beijing.

Regardless of the terms of the reward that Chen Chang put forth, it was he that Chen Chang wanted and it was he that Chen Chang would follow. He had no desire to lead Chen Chang and the others anywhere near his village or his friends. Besides, there was the evil he'd felt in the forest. Its presence still weighed on him. He wondered when he would again feel that unwanted force. He knew that one day he would come face to face with the evil energy and he had to be ready to defeat it.

There was also a chance they'd take Pei Ke hostage, but regardless of what the reward said, Liu didn't think the boy was in any danger. They would only use him to get to Liu.

Liu knew Pei Ke was still trying to decide what to do, but he had little doubt what the outcome would be. The matching of the coins would bring him instant wealth, but Liu was confident Pei Ke would not take the treasure and the wealth of the lands. He felt he had instilled in the young man enough dedication and curiosity about Chinese internal martial arts and Traditional Chinese Medicine for him to forsake the comforts and pleasures of money, as Liu had done earlier in his life.

He suspected Pei Ke was only a day, maybe two day's journey behind him. The real question was whether Pei Ke would take the road to the left or the one to the right. Either road would bring Pei Ke to Beijing. Liu realized that if what the man he'd killed told the truth there were indeed bounty hunters lining the road to Beijing. The road to the right would probably be safer. At the same time, Liu himself would provide the best protection, not to mention the fact the road to the left would offer many opportunities for Pei Ke to learn and grow.

Liu paused and closed his eyes. He meditated first on the road to the left and then on Pei Ke. He subconsciously called out to Pei Ke to take the road to the left. He felt the energy concept of taking the road to the left leave his body and travel at lightning speed back down the road. At first, he wondered if Pei Ke would experience the energy being sent his way. But after a couple of minutes, he realized the energy had arrived at its destination and Pei Ke would make the right choice. Nodding to himself, he continued on his way.

A little way down the road eyes once again watched him. Liu briefly looked into the forest, but could not see them; he could only sense their presence.

# CHAPTER TWO

Pei Ke walked past the two monks sweeping the cobblestone walkway. They were typical of the monks that he had seen before at the temple. It was obvious they took pleasure in their activity as they smiled with almost an inner smile of peace and contentment. Pei Ke knew that their spiritual training prepared them to be part of the continuous life cycle exemplified in Taoist and Buddhist traditions.

From his training with Liu Bin, he appreciated that the Yin and Yang of their lives was intertwined with the Yin and Yang of all things within nature. The inhabitants of the temple were indeed in balance with their environment. This harmony came not only from the daily activities they performed, but also from their regular and intense meditation. Each morning, afternoon, and evening, they were called together to bring the whole temple into a unison of thought and activities. This was different from other temples where prayer and meditation were only twice a day. This temple was unique and Pei Ke knew it from what he had experienced with the Abbot.

His mind was made up and out of respect for the Abbot and monks at the temple, he needed to convey his decision rather than just walk away. After all, he would not have made this decision without the Abbot's help.

He was excited about what he had decided. He had vacillated about his choices to the point he was unable to make a decision. His emotions were so overwhelming that none of the energy could flow properly until the Abbot opened up his spiritual gates allowing the free flow of energy. He remembered the Abbot touching various acupuncture points on his head and body. He felt a sinking experience and total relaxation of mind and body until he fell asleep.

He guessed he slept for at least four hours. It was one of the deepest and most calming experiences he had ever had. Every muscle relaxed to the point where there was no tension anywhere in his body—so much so that he did not feel any of his physical body. It was a state of complete and total relaxation. He wondered if Liu with his Ancient Wisdom had taught the Abbot this Ancient Knowledge?

His teacher, Liu Bin, knew much about the ways of energy and martial arts. He distinctly remembered dreaming about the amulet around his neck, and what it meant for him and others. His dreams switched between his teacher and the beautiful girls Mei Li and Hua Yee who he had recently met. Every time he thought of either one of the girls he felt a stirring deep within.

Before the Abbot calmed his spirit he was too agitated to make a decision, but things were different now. The dreaming process seemed to place everything that happened to him into pockets in his conscious and subconscious mind giving him a much needed clarity of thought to see what he needed to accomplish with his life. He was excited and for the first time since his parents died, he felt highly focused. He needed to find the Abbot.

He knew the Abbot would again ask him to make a decision to stay and receive the Liu family treasure, or give up the amulet and search for Liu. He didn't understand why he had to give up the amulet if he searched for his teacher. He needed to tell the Abbot that he was going to look for Liu and not give up the amulet. He didn't know why Liu left him behind but he was going to find out. Liu had entrusted the amulet to him and he was going to safeguard it until Liu himself told him differently.

As he walked into the Abbot's office he was met by one of the attending monks. Initial greetings were exchanged between the two of them

"Is the Abbot in?" asked Pei Ke.

"No, he has gone out to be with one of the members of the temple. He will be back tomorrow."

———————

Mei Li usually focused on the tasks at hand, accomplishing what was needed to be done. She had the ability to make things happen and her father, Wei Ken De, relied on her ability. Since his wife had passed she had assumed ever increasing responsibilities both within the household and the business Wei Ken De owned. He was grooming his daughter to one day take over the family business. He and his deceased wife had built the business from humble beginnings to a very successful enterprise.

He noticed that recently her focus was intermittent and activities which should have been done immediately were being put off till another day. It was obvious she was concentrating on something other than what was expected of her. A couple of times he found her staring off into empty space with a slight grin or smile. Whatever was capturing her attention, it was pleasing. He was not sure where or when the change took place, but it seemed to start when Liu Bin, his martial arts teacher, visited with them. Maybe Liu had mentioned something to her. Whatever it was he knew he would eventually find out. He trusted the Universal Energy would be in his favor and protect his daughter.

———————

Hua Yee could not shake the deep seated hatred for those who had killed her parents and most of her relatives. The only family remaining was her uncle Liu Bin, her younger brother and sisters, and their cousins. She was furious when she found out one or more of the assailants had escaped. It was not her uncle's fault. He had done what was expected of him. There were just too many of them for him to deal with them all at the same time.

She was underage and knew she had to stay with friends of the family until she came of age. She promised her dead parents and the spirit of her ancestors that one day she would hunt down the remaining assailants and kill them. For now, she had to wait and bide her time.

She had met Pei Ke, her uncle's student, and found him exceedingly handsome. She made a mental note to speak with her uncle about getting married. She would be of age next year and her uncle needed to find her a suitable husband. Pei Ke would be quite suitable. Surely her uncle would agree with her. She fantasized giving herself up to Pei Ke.

———————

Pei Ke headed from the temple to Mr. Wu's house. He made a mental note to visit with the Abbot the next day. He knew exactly what to do. The key was Mr. Wu who he hoped would guide him and give him counsel in his decision. He thought he knew where Liu was going, but he needed to be sure before he tried to catch up with him.

As he walked, he considered the paths he'd taken that had led him here. He had been studying Traditional Chinese Medicine and Chinese internal martial arts with Master Liu Bin for over two years. In those initial days with Liu, they started each morning with a Qi Gong or martial arts workout. He always looked forward to these lessons in martial arts. The training set the tone for how he felt for the rest of the day.

On the rare occasion that he missed a workout, he noticed he didn't feel quite as good the rest of the day. It was almost like an addiction, he thought, though in this case a good and healthy one. That routine had almost come to a halt, however, when Liu had received the message supposedly from his older brother.

In response to the note, Liu had abruptly decided to leave and Pei Ke had asked to join him. Together, they had travelled north towards Liu's ancestral home, uncertain what they would find there. During the three-week journey, Pei Ke learned a tremendous amount about martial arts and Chinese medicine. Each day, from sunrise to sunset, Pei Ke had listened to his teacher lecture on the various aspects of Traditional Chinese Medicine. He watched as his teacher helped others with various health care issues. Of course, there had been a fair amount of fighting as well, as Chen Su's men had tried to prevent Liu Bin from reaching his home and interfering with Chen Su's invasion. Pei Ke had had the opportunity to watch a true martial arts master in action.

Now, he walked briskly towards Mr. Wu's home. He was thankful for all he had learned and now realized he missed those daily lessons. Liu was like a father, guiding him towards his destiny.

His thoughts shifted to Wei Ken De's house. He and Liu had visited the house on their journey north. Wei Ken De was one of Liu's top martial arts students and it was there that he met Mei Li. Even though the visit was brief, it was clear that she liked him as much as he liked her. He instantly knew that she would be the perfect wife. But he was poor and she came from an upper class merchant family. His thoughts turned to the amulet and what it possibly meant for him. He could be rich but would that make a difference to her.

On the other hand, Hua Yee was also beautiful. Just as pretty as Mei Li and most certainly someone he would be proud to have as his wife. If the present circumstances were different he could easily find himself attracted to her. She had made it clear that she'd like to see him again. It was a bold move on her part, but he definitely intended to respond to it. Would she also make the perfect wife? He knew it was possible, but he wasn't sure now was the right time.

He passed through the same rise that he and Liu had passed weeks before on their initial visit to Wu's house. He remembered the emotional meeting between Liu and his niece Hua Yee when the door had opened and she'd run to Liu in tears. This scene was firmly etched in his mind. He could not think about that meeting without thinking about another night, when Liu had taken revenge on Chen Su for slaughtering his family.

Pei Ke shuddered. To his continual discomfort, he had accidently played a minor but significant role in the retribution. He had never killed a man before and even though Chen Su's men had killed Liu's family for their land and fortune, Pei Ke never again wanted to be part of taking another's life. It was a conflict and contradiction. He loved studying martial arts because it gave him a sense of security and power; however, he loathed the outcome of what he was training himself to do.

As he approached Mr. Wu's walled estate, two guards appeared from almost nowhere to challenge him. He recognized one of the guards from his first visit. The guard recognized him as well and bowed slightly. Pei Ke returned the bow.

While he waited, word was sent to Mr. Wu and after a few minutes the door opened slowly. Hua Yee emerged smiling. Pei Ke was struck by the contrast between his first visit and now. The first visit was tears and this visit was a show of happiness. The tears of the first visit were a combination of her parents being maliciously killed and being reunited with her only living adult relative.

He could tell that she was restraining herself as she submitted to etiquette and paused in the door as Mr. Wu came and walked out to greet him. Pei Ke noticed her watching him and he felt his heart flutter. She was indeed beautiful and he briefly wondered what life would be like with her as his wife.

Hua Yee stared at Pei Ke. She had known deep in her heart he would return. She didn't realize it would be so soon. She must find time to be alone with him.

Nothing had changed at Wu's house, but nothing was expected to change. Pei Ke surmised that the grieving period was over and that Hua Yee and the other children had been accepted into Wu's home as his own.

The relationship between the Wu and Liu families went deep, spanning more than a couple of generations, each helping the other without any question or challenge. Pei Ke knew that such a relationship was invaluable, especially in times such as these.

He bowed low to Mr. Wu, who returned the bow to a depth expressing his station in life.

"Welcome back," said Mr. Wu. "Please come in and have some tea with us. Have you eaten?"

"Thank you. Some tea would be especially good. The day is still chilly and I have just come from the temple."

"Come in, then, it is warmer inside. We can talk when you have had some tea and feel warmer."

Pei Ke followed Mr. Wu and Hua Yee through the outer courtyard and into his house. Even though he had been there numerous times and had stayed with Mr. Wu just recently, it seemed like a long time had passed since he was last there. Something in him had changed.

Wu led them into the sitting room and motioned for him to sit down. He sat in one chair. Wu sat in another, and Hua Yee sat close to her adopted uncle. As she sat down, Pei Ke noticed the braided string around her neck, which he assumed was her part of the amulet. He remembered the story of the amulet and how he came to acquire it from Master Liu. What he didn't know was whether or not Hua Yee was aware of the significance of what she had around her neck.

The three sat in silence for a moment. It was obvious to Pei Ke that Wu wanted him to speak first.

"Mr. Wu, thank you for seeing me. Master Liu has left the temple, but I do not know where he has gone. I asked the Abbot, but he would not tell me. I have decided to follow Liu, but I need to know where he has gone. I am guessing he has told you."

"Yes," said Wu. "Liu told me before he departed where he was going, just as he told me you would be coming to talk to me. He told me you would have decided what you want to do with your life. Is that true?"

Pei Ke was startled and didn't know what to say. How had Master Liu known he'd come to Wu for help? He looked at Hua Yee. She had a faint smile on her face. He wondered what she knew about Liu and where he was going. He was grasping for words when Wu spoke again.

"Your teacher confided in me just before you two left to go to the temple. He asked me to keep this information in confidence. He also shared it with Hua Yee, and she knows not to share it with anyone else. Of course, the other children being very young have no idea where he is going. They will remain here and I will take care of them."

The servants brought in the tea and Hua Yee poured it for the two men. She was about to pour some for herself when Wu spoke.

"Hua Yee, please excuse us. I would like to speak with Pei Ke in private."

Pei Ke could see the disappointment in her face as she put the tea pot on the tray. She looked at him for a fraction of a second, smiled, and then turned to Wu.

"Of course, Uncle Wu. If there is anything you need, please just call me."

Pei Ke smiled at her and when he looked back at Wu, the old man was staring at him.

"Will you check on the children?" Wu said to Hua Yee, as he continued looking at Pei Ke. "They are on the other side of the house. Stay with them and make sure they have something constructive to do. I will call for you when we are done."

"Yes, Uncle."

After Hua Yee left, Wu continued to gaze at Pei Ke. Finally he cleared his throat and spoke.

"As you know there is a very close relationship between myself and the Liu family. Our families have been through much together. They have helped me immeasurably and I am indebted to them."

Pei Ke nodded at this. Wu continued.

"Hua Yee is entrusted to my care and I will do whatever is necessary to protect her. She is still young but is coming of age. It seems clear to me that you are also concerned with her best interest and would do anything to protect her. Am I correct?"

"Yes, definitely," said Pei Ke.

Clearly, Wu knew of their attraction, but Pei Ke wondered if he knew what Hua Yee had said to him. It almost sounded like Wu was going to give Pei Ke his blessing to court Hua Yee and for a split second, he wavered in his decision to follow Liu Bin. Was Wu telling him something? He didn't know what to say.

"Pei Ke, you have come here to find out where Liu has gone. Is that correct?"

"Yes, Mr. Wu, that is correct."

"What do you intend to do?"

"I would like to continue my studies with Liu and learn as much as possible from him. He has an extensive knowledge of Chinese martial arts and Traditional Chinese Medicine. I would like to learn all that he knows."

"Do you realize his knowledge comes from many years of study from numerous teachers? This is in addition to his personal readings and studies. It would be impossible for anyone to acquire this knowledge quickly. And so I am wondering how long you are willing to study with him, and what you plan to do after you have finished your studies?"

Pei Ke knew he wanted to continue studying with Liu and to do so he needed to find Liu. He also knew he had an attraction for both Hua Yee and Mei Li. He just hadn't thought through the process of what he was going to do later in life. Was Wu trying to get him to think through this process?

"I definitely want to find Teacher and continue studying with him," he said a little impatiently. "I have not decided what I will do later in life. It is customary to settle down, get married, and have a family; but, I have not thought that far ahead."

"And if you couldn't find Liu Bin?"

"Honestly, Mr. Wu, the thought never crossed my mind."

Wu nodded slowly and narrowed his eyes as though considering something. He didn't speak for some time and Pei Ke waited anxiously for his reply.

"Pei Ke," he finally said, "why don't you stay here for the night and we can discuss it more tomorrow. I have to go into the village to get some things. While I am away give some thought to staying here on a permanent basis. You will get to know the area better and help look after the Liu estate until he returns. When Liu returns then you and he can plan your future."

Pei Ke nodded his understanding and murmured his thanks, though he did so quietly to hide his disappointment. He wanted to be on his way, but he could not offend Wu. That night Pei Ke thought about Hua Yee and the possibility of staying on with Mr. Wu. He fell asleep quite uncertain as to what to do. He felt Mr. Wu was putting pressure on him to stay.

# CHAPTER THREE

In the morning they had breakfast together, separate from the rest of the family.

"Pei Ke, have some more tea."

Pei Ke picked up the warm teapot and poured some tea for Wu, then for himself. He'd already had two cups of tea. It was good, but he found himself thinking about the tea he'd shared with Liu Bin at the inn their first night of travel. It had been much better. Better than any tea Pei Ke had ever had. That all seemed like years ago.

"Pei Ke, I know you are aware that Hua Yee comes of age soon."

The statement caught Pei Ke off guard. He needed to be careful how he responded.

"Yes, I am aware that she is coming of age."

"Last night you mentioned the possibility of some day getting married and having a family? Is there someone special you have met and might want to marry?"

From the corner of his eye Pei Ke caught the slight movement of Hua Yee's clothes at the entrance to the room. She was obviously hiding behind the wall and a small part of her dress inadvertently had passed into the opening for a fraction of a second.

"My parents are deceased and no arrangements had been made between my family and another for marriage, so I am free to marry anyone."

Pei Ke looked carefully at Wu studying his expressions trying to read the older man's mind before he continued. He was certain Wu was in the process of making a decision. What Pei Ke said next would be important in that decision process. Here we are two men trying to read each other's minds before making a decision. At the same time, Pei Ke wanted to send a message to Hua Yee.

"There is a girl I recently met who is beautiful and I am attracted to her, but I am poor and my status in life is not in keeping with her status."

"Liu has put a lot of trust in you," said Wu. "He speaks highly of you for your enthusiasm, dedication, and honesty. As I mentioned last night, if you would like to stay here I can make arrangements for you to work and get settled down. If you follow after Liu how are you going to support yourself?"

"I am willing to work for my meals and lodging."

"If you leave here will you be going directly to find Liu?"

*There must be a reason Wu is asking me this question*, thought Pei Ke. *Maybe he is going to send a message to Liu and let Liu know what I am doing.*

"No, I want to go see Wei Ken De, one of Liu's senior students. We stayed with him before coming here. It is a day's journey south. He will be concerned about Liu since he knew why Teacher was traveling north. It is only right for me to keep him informed of the events surrounding the Liu family."

Wu looked at Pei Ke for the longest time before speaking. He was digesting the information he had gleaned from the young man.

"Liu told me to tell you he has gone to Beijing. You can find him in one of the old Hu Tong areas near the West Gate. Most people are familiar with this area. You will know what to do and where to go once you get there."

"Have you been there?" asked Pei Ke.

"No, I have not been to Beijing. Very few people here, other than your teacher, have been outside of this area. Everything we need and want can be found here, so there is no need to explore other areas. Don't you think this is an ideal place to live and bring up a family?"

Pei Ke nodded slowly.

"Yes, this place is ideal. Maybe one day, I can settle down here, and as you say start a family."

"Have you said good-bye to the Abbot at the temple?"

"No, I have not. He was not in when I went to see him. I will visit with him later. I have not said good-bye to Hua Yee. With your permission I would like to say good-bye to her."

"While you are getting your things, I will find her. She must be with the children."

Pei Ke went to the room he had stayed in the night before. He only had a coat to pick up. As he entered the room he saw Hua Yee standing in the middle of the room. She looked quite beautiful.

"I hope you don't think it too bold of me to be here," she said. "I know Uncle Wu would not allow us to speak together alone. I just wanted to again thank you for helping Uncle Liu Bin avenge the death of my family. I am deeply indebted to you."

Pei Ke looked at her and thought about what had happened to her family and what Liu had done. What he himself had done. It made him angry to think that Chen Su's son had escaped. He wondered if their paths would cross again one day. He wondered what he would do if they did.

Hua Yee smiled at him, then turned her gaze downwards. Pei Ke felt a warmth course through his body. He'd experienced this before, but with a different woman, a woman he was leaving to see now.

"When will you come back to see me—excuse me—to see us again?"

Pei Ke's heart beat even faster. It was obvious she liked him and wanted to see him again. He was going to say something when Hua Yee again smiled. He returned the smile.

He reached into the opening of his shirt and lifted the hidden amulet just enough so Hua Yee could see the outline of the broken coin. She stared at the amulet and uttered a slight gasp of recognition. Her hand went immediately to her chest to feel the amulet hidden underneath her clothes. She didn't know what to say, but understood the implication of Pei Ke having the coin. She hoped that in the immediate future she and Pei Ke would one day be brought together. Maybe the coins would be the catalyst for bringing them together.

She smiled shyly as she walked past him. He recognized the slight smell of lavender. She looked deep into his eyes. Her clothes gently brushed up against his pants.

"I must go now," said Hua Yee. "Uncle Wu will be looking for me. I will anxiously be awaiting your return. We can talk more when I see you again. Stay safe and say hello to uncle."

As she walked through the door she briefly looked back and smiled. Pei Ke stood there for a couple of moments not knowing what to do. His heart was beating fast. He walked out of the room and went to the sitting room.

Wu was waiting for him.

"Hua Yee must be helping the children outside," said Wu. "I have asked the servants to look for her."

Just then Hua Yee entered the room. She walked over to Wu.

"Did you call for me, uncle?"

"Yes. Pei Ke has decided to go to Beijing and find your uncle," said Wu. "It is still early in the day and he wants to get a quick start on his journey."

Pei Ke bowed to Wu and he returned the bow. For a brief moment Hua Yee and Pei Ke exchanged glances. She bowed as was the custom. Wu walked Pei Ke out the door across the estate courtyard to the main gate.

They exchanged pleasantries before Pei Ke turned and walked past the ever present guards. Pei Ke again wondered if he had made the right decision. An alliance through marriage with Hua Yee would be possible with Liu's blessing. His status in life and wealth beyond his dreams would be instantly possible.

After he'd walked for a few minutes he turned to look back at Wu's estate. No one was there. Even the guards were gone. Again he wondered if he made the right decision. He looked in the direction of Beijing, then Wu's house, and then south towards the road leading to Wei Ken De's house.

He walked back to the village and went directly to the temple. He bowed recognition to the monks who were present. He stood for a few moments in front of the statue of Kuan Yin and then knelt down and prayed as his mother had taught him to pray when he was a child.

When he was finished with his prayers he rose, turned, and was startled to see the Abbot standing behind him. He was not more than five feet from him.

"Have a safe trip," said the Abbot. "Say hello to Master Liu for us. Be sure and tell him Kuan Yin is looking over everything and everybody."

Pei Ke wondered how the Abbot knew he was going to Beijing to visit with Liu. He was about to ask the Abbot, but the Abbot suddenly turned and walked away before he could ask the question. The Abbot never looked back. There was finality to the encounter. It was eerie the way it ended. He wanted to thank the Abbot for what he had done, but the Abbot just kept on walking away.

Pei Ke shrugged the encounter off as he walked out of the temple. He looked around the small village. There were a few people on the dusty streets. They seemed to have a purpose to their lives as they moved around.

Pei Ke mentally said good bye to the village, not knowing when he would be back, and headed for Liu's ancestral home. He wanted to pay his respects at the graves of his teacher's family.

He remembered the way to the valley. As he went over the crest of the mountain, he stopped at the same place Liu had stopped weeks before to look at the peaceful valley and its idealistic surroundings. He thought of Hua Yee. It was possible this could very well be his someday. He could see himself and Hua Yee happily married in this peaceful valley.

As he descended the mountain, he thought he saw movement in the distant trees. He stopped to watch the trail. He didn't know if his eyes were playing tricks on him or if there really had been some movement off in the distance.

Sometime later, he entered the same gate he and Liu had entered when they previously arrived at Liu's ancestral home. Nothing had changed since they were last there. After quickly walking around the compound he went outside the gates to the graves and made sure they had not been disturbed. Everything looked in order. He bowed to Liu's brother's grave and mentally made a note to tell Liu the gravesites were undisturbed.

Next, he went back to the house and visited the various rooms Liu had previously shown him, including the room Liu had used as a child. As he entered the sitting room, he scanned the room. Everything was in its original place, just as they had left it weeks earlier. He went to the secret hiding place and paused for a moment. Should he check to see if the area had been disturbed?

Liu had made no attempt to keep the location secret from him. He'd seen how Liu had gained access by removing the books and pushing against the panel. Finally, Pei Ke did the same and the door opened. The sword and knife that had been there before were missing. Had Liu or had someone else taken the items?

Pei Ke stayed the night in Liu's ancestral home. He slept in the same room that Liu slept in as a child. As he fell asleep his thoughts were with his teacher. Where was he? What was he doing?

The next morning he woke at first light to begin the trip to Wei Ken De's home. He took one final look around the property to firmly etch it in his mind. After closing the gate he headed back in the direction he had come. Occasionally, he would stop and look out over the expansive valley. At the summit, he took one final look. Off in the distance he again saw unusual movement in the trees. He stared at the location for many minutes, then finally turned and headed away from the summit. A cold wind blew forcefully against his body and he sensed someone watching him from afar.

# CHAPTER FOUR

Pei Ke's trip south to Wei Ken De's home was uneventful. To conserve time, he had skipped that morning's martial arts practice. Instead he alternated between running and brisk walking. He never would have been able to keep up the pace without the previous training he had received from Liu. As a result, he managed to arrive while there was still light in the sky.

His thoughts during most of the trip vacillated between Hua Yee, Mei Li, and Liu Bin. Both of the girls were beautiful and each one of them presented with different attributes he found pleasing. Continuing the blood line of his ancestors was important and each one he felt could easily do that for him.

His major concerns of money and martial arts would be solved with the union of either one of them. One day in the not too distant future he needed to make a decision.

He pulled the string and listened for the ring of the bell. Moments later, he heard the familiar sound of the bolt sliding open and exposing the peep hole. The man behind must have recognized Pei Ke for he was told to wait for a few moments. After what felt like an eternity, the door slowly opened and the same man who had greeted him before motioned for him to enter.

Pei Ke was led into the house and told to sit. He took the same seat he'd taken weeks before. Everything was as it had been before.

When Wei Ken De entered the room, Pei Ke frowned inwardly that Mei Li wasn't with him, but he did not outwardly express his feelings. Instead, he stood up and bowed in respect to one of Liu's top students. Wei Ken De acknowledged the greeting.

"Where is Master Liu?" asked Wei Ken De. "Is he all right?"

"Master Liu is fine. He has gone to Beijing. I have come to tell you what has happened since we were last here. I thought you, being one of his senior students, should know."

"Sit down," said Wei Ken De. Pei Ke felt as he had the last time he'd been here: intimidated by this powerful personality.

Pei Ke looked at Wei Ken De for a moment trying to decide how to start. There was so much to tell and he wanted to get it all in the correct order.

"Well, speak up. What has happened?"

The tone of voice was unsettling. It made Pei Ke feel a little intimidated. He couldn't discern if the mood of Wei Ken De was just harshness or anticipation of what Pei Ke was about to relate.

He started to relate the details of what had happened but no more than five minutes into the story, there was a knock on the door. Wei Ken De got up and opened the door, hesitated for a brief second, then walked back to his chair. Mei Li followed.

Pei Ke stood up, and they exchanged courtesies. He was careful not to look at her too long, or to smile too much. He did not want to let on that he was really there to see Mei Li.

For the next hour, he related to Wei Ken De and Mei Li what had happened, including the revenge Liu had taken on those who had killed most of his family. He even included the small but relevant part he had played. Mei Li, as expected, did not utter one word but looked at Pei Ke with ever increasing fondness.

She had thought about Pei Ke often since he and Liu had abruptly left weeks before. She wished they had stayed. She wanted Liu to stay so she could study more Hsing-Yi Chuan from the famous master. She wanted Pei Ke to stay because his presence touched something special in her mind and body. She thought maybe he was the one. She never dreamed he would be back so soon. There were things she had wanted to say to him before but couldn't. Now he was back and she would not miss her chance again.

Wei Ken De, on the other hand, had many questions and the need for Pei Ke to elaborate on certain facts of the encounter. One of the details Pei Ke omitted was the information on the coin and the matching of the coin parts to form a whole coin indicating how the Liu family wealth could be distributed. As he spoke about being in the temple, he subconsciously felt the coin around his neck. It was still safe.

It was getting late when Pei Ke finally finished answering all of Wei Ken De's questions.

"What are you going to do now since Teacher has gone to Beijing?" asked Wei Ken De.

Mei Li held her breath, waiting for his answer. *Is this too good to be true?* she thought.

"I want to continue my studies of Chinese internal martial arts and Traditional Chinese Medicine."

Wei Ken Da nodded. Pei Ke interpreted this as an approval from Wei Ken Da.

"It is getting late," he said. "Why don't you stay here for the evening? You can have dinner with us. I will instruct the servants to add one more for dinner and to prepare a place for you to sleep."

"Thank you," said Pei Ke.

"Thank you for going out of your way to bring this information to me. As you know, I hold our teacher in high esteem. I knew his journey back home was going to be difficult but did not know it was going to be that difficult. You have done well to keep him company and help him. By the way, do you carry any coins with you?"

Pei Ke was startled by the question. He was sure Mei Li could tell there was a change in his composure. Did Wei Ken De know the story of the coins? He was sure he did not. It had to be just a coincidence that Wei Ken De asked him.

"Yes, I have a few coins, but not much. I really do not need a lot."

Wei Ken De nodded again, ignoring any indications he saw of Pei Ke's discomfort.

"Mei Li will give you some coins for your trip. Give what you do not need to Teacher. He may need the money while he is in Beijing."

"May I be so bold as to ask a question?"

Mei Li's heart skipped a beat. A slight blush came to her face. Many thoughts went racing through her head. She smiled and gazed downward in anticipation of the question Pei Ke was going to ask.

"What is your question?"

"May I speak with you in private?"

Wei Ken De looked at Pei Ke and then at Mei Li. He could see the blush on his daughter's face.

"Whatever you want to ask me you can ask while Mei Li is here. We have no secrets between us."

# CHAPTER FIVE

As he looked back on the event, how he survived was truly a miracle. Enough poison from the King Cobra had been injected into his leg to kill two ordinary people, but Bao was not an ordinary person. He was stronger than most men and conditioned for hardship. His life had always been in some type of turmoil and many times it bordered on the not so legal side of an activity. This was no exception. The attack on the Liu ancestral compound was to bring him some needed money and maybe a cut into the fantastic wealth of the Liu family.

It had been some time since he had been at the Liu estate. He remembered putting all thoughts of wealth out of his mind. He had focused only on his survival. He had acted quickly. He had heard of men who had been bit by this type of snake—a King Cobra—and few of them ever survived.

He had survived the ordeal through shear ingenuity and fortitude. As soon as he had been bit, he took his knife and made two deep cuts next to the bite area. These were not superficial cuts, but deep cuts. He hoped that if enough venom escaped through the incision he would survive the bite.

He remembered putting a tourniquet on the wound and forcing out as much blood as he could, hoping it forced the remaining toxin out of his body.

The snake attack was quite unexpected. He had only seen a cobra once before and it was in the south. He knew they didn't exist this far north. It had to have been imported. A cobra was a good choice for its raised body and flared head instilled fear in everyone.

He reflected on how the situation had developed. After he and the other two men entered the underground hiding place through the overhead entrance to the corral water trough, the snakes had attacked. Everyone had been bitten at least once by the three snakes, and all thoughts of continuing their search for the Liu ancestral treasure were abandoned. They now concentrated on their survival.

The broken ladder leading down into the hideout meant almost certain death. After their first two attempts to get out failed, Bao went over to the door where the swords were found.

He remembered taking off all his clothes and cutting everything into strips, twisting the pieces together into sections, and then tying the sections together to make a rope. He tied one end of the makeshift rope to the only long piece of broken ladder that remained, and threw it upwards towards the opening, hoping the piece of ladder would catch on the lip of the hole.

After the fourth attempt, it caught on the outside of the trough and Bao started to climb up the makeshift rope. Just as his hand grasped the inner edge of the opening, the makeshift rope started to unravel. With adrenaline flowing, he thrust his other hand upwards and used all his remaining strength to pull himself up and over the edge to safety.

He had looked back into the hole and was about to go for help when he noticed a small beam of diffused light coming from a crack in the underground wall. He closed the cover to the trough and sat down on the cold ground as ever increasing wind blew over his naked body. He heard pleas from the two still in the underground hole but he ignored them. He sealed their fate, but he now knew where the treasure was hidden, and only he knew. Even if the two accomplices' in the hole discovered the light, they would be dead by morning. He now needed to concentrate on his own survival. The poison from the King Cobra was taking its toll on his body.

---

Chen Su and his son Chen Chang had found Bao outside the corral gate lying naked on the ground. They noticed the deep cut marks and assumed

Bao had been in a fight. Chen Su was baffled he could not find the other two men he sent to check the corral. He brought enough men to make sure that the Liu family would be killed all at once. He kept track of who he brought, how many he brought, and exactly what each was to do in the attack. He was even more baffled to find Bao unconscious and naked. He did not know who had attacked Bao, but did not want to stay behind and find out. Whoever it was would surely notify the local authorities. He did not want him and his men to be around when they came. He assumed the other two were either dead or had run away as he and his men took Bao and headed out the gate.

# CHAPTER SIX

Liu found a high place along the road with a beautiful view of the mountains. Looking far into the distance, he was sure he could see the peaks close to his ancestral home.

He thought of the last three months. The strange message he'd received at the temple requesting his return home. The subsequent travels with Pei Ke as they'd traveled from his residence at the temple northwards.

He reflected on the violent attacks he'd encountered on the trip and his ability even at his age to have successfully defended himself and Pei Ke. The trip had not been all bad. He had stopped many times to visit with long-time friends. It was at one of his stops that he spent time with Wei Ken De. He had many other students over the years, but Wei Ken De was the most accomplished and the most loyal of all of them, allowing him to bear the distinction of "inner door" student.

He grew sad as he considered the outcome of the journey. His family, with the exception of Hua Yee, the children, and a servant boy had been massacred. He had taken revenge and that memory saddened him even more. Doing so had violated one of the tenets he had held sacred. All life was precious, and he had violated those teachings by killing in revenge. And now he had once again violated what he had taught others.

It was because of this that he was now taking this journey in the twilight of his life. He needed to see some old friends, friends he trusted, who had taken different and more traditional roads in their lives. He had taken a road few had traveled. He had done this with almost everything in his life.

But was the less-traveled road with its discipline and monastic life really worth it? He felt that it was, but in light of what had happened at his ancestral home he needed to see the opposite. It was like Yin and Yang. For him to see the truth of his decision, he needed to see it's opposite.

His thoughts turned to his father who had initially trained him in the family martial arts. His mother had been responsible in part for teaching him the finer things in life, such as calligraphy, painting, and poetry. He had a good life as a child and though he had chosen a different life as an adult, he wanted for nothing. The years of hard training and study had given him the ability to do with much less than others. In fact, he eschewed the good life that others strived for. His good life was his interaction with the Universal Energy of nature.

Liu felt the chill of the winter wind and the warmth of the sun; the warmth balancing out the cold. Suddenly, he sensed a shift in the surrounding energy. He knew instantly this was a good shift. Pei Ke was coming.

# CHAPTER SEVEN

Pei Ke rounded the corner and saw Liu seated on a rock staring at the distant mountains. Pei Ke slowly walked up to his teacher and bowed low in respect. Liu looked up and gazed deeply into his student's eyes. Pei Ke felt the intensity of his teacher's eye contact. It seemed as if Liu was looking deep into his very soul, looking for an answer to a question.

"Pei Ke, what took you so long? I have been waiting here for you."

"Master, how did you know I was coming?"

"You only had three choices. The energy of learning was greater than the energy of romance and money."

Pei Ke blushed as he realized Liu knew of his affection for Mei Li. He wondered if he knew he also had similar affection for his niece Hua Yee.

"How did you know I…"

"Your mind was in turmoil over the choices. That is why I had you visit with the Abbot. I asked him to clear your mind so you would not agonize over whether or not you made the right decision."

"What if I had made one of the other choices?" asked Pei Ke.

"Do you feel sad about your decision?"

"No. Absolutely not."

"Then don't worry about it. You made what you felt was the right decision. Your decision does not preclude you from other things later, whereas, one of the other decisions would have led you down paths precluding further learning on your part."

Pei Ke thought of his last conversation with the Abbot before he'd left the temple to follow Liu.

Liu motioned for Pei Ke to sit next to him on the boulder. They sat in silence, both deep in thought. Pei Ke was thinking about his decision and what lay ahead for him. Was he going to travel with Liu forever or was this to be a short trip?

Liu was happy that Pei Ke had made the right decision to eschew the riches of life and to continue his studies of martial arts and medicine. He now needed to push his student even harder for him to progress to the next level of mastery.

Pei Ke was about to ask Liu a question when his teacher said, "Pei Ke it is time for us to move on. We are headed to Beijing. It will take us a few days to get there. The night air will be very cold tonight with possible snow and I want to get to the inn a few miles down the road."

"Before you arrived did you see anyone on the road?"

"No, Master."

"When you came to the fork in the road, how did you know to take the road to the left?"

"The energy felt good. I was kind of pulled in that direction."

"Good," said Liu.

"Master, after I left the temple, I went to see Mr. Wu who told me where you would be. I also went to your ancestral home to pay respect to your family and to make sure that everything was undisturbed. I took the liberty of checking on the secret place where you had the sword and knife. They were gone."

"Yes," said Liu. "I have moved them to Mr. Wu's house."

"After leaving your home I went to see Wei Ken De to tell him what had happened since we were last there. He gave me some coins to give to you."

"Pei Ke, you did well," said Liu. "Hold on to the coins for me."

Liu smiled, stood up, and started walking east along the road. Pei Ke quickly followed—teacher and student were once again united. Liu sensed no danger and smiled to himself. Pei Ke held his question for another time and another place.

As night approached they stayed at a small inn secluded in a pine forest, just off the road. Liu had stayed here many years previously and unless someone had built a new inn, he knew this was the only available lodging for many miles. Anyone on the road had to either stay at the inn or brave the elements for the night. It was going to be a cold evening and Liu was happy they were going to spend it in comfort.

# CHAPTER EIGHT

Liu and Pei Ke had been traveling for two days when they approached a series of descending rice paddies. The paddies were situated on both sides of the narrow road. One paddy followed another in such a manner that it appeared far off into the distance that the road was going to be squeezed by the paddies.

As they walked, the farmers in the paddies looked up to watch the two men walking and then looked off into the distance. One farmer looking in their direction they were going would be a non-issue, but when most of the farmers in the fields started doing the same Liu stopped and looked at Pei Ke.

"Master, why are we stopping?"

"Did you notice that when most of the farmers saw us they looked down the road? Clearly they know something we do not and the Universal Energy has an evil taint to it here. I fear there is something evil ahead."

Pei Ke looked down the road but could see nothing. As they were talking one of the farmers beckoned for them to come over to the side of the road. Liu and Pei Ke met the farmer at the edge of the rice paddy.

"You may want to reconsider going down that road," said the farmer. "The local gang has been drinking all night. They are harassing not only us villagers but also any travelers on the road. If you have anything of value, you might want to turn back; they will surely take it from you."

"How many of them are there?" asked Liu.

"I am not certain but there are usually four or five hanging out together. When they get like this, there's no telling what they'll do."

"Have you called the local magistrate to put an end to their behavior?" asked Liu.

The man shook his head sadly.

"It will do no good. One of the boys has a very influential father. He is quite elderly and has no control of his son. When we've tried to talk to him about it, he denies there's a problem. When we mentioned it to the magistrate, he dismisses it as the minor pranks of young boys. Most of us have decided to leave the situation alone as long as their activities are not too flagrant."

"Have they been drinking recently?" asked Liu

"Yes they were drinking last night and are still drinking today."

"Thank you," said Liu.

He bowed politely and turned back to the road and started walking.

"Pei Ke, are you coming?"

"Yes, Master. Shouldn't we look for another road?"

"I don't know of another way to get to Beijing. Of course, I could walk through the rice paddies and climb over the hills. I think it is easier to just continue walking."

"What if the gang causes us problems?" asked Pei Ke.

"Let's look at it from a positive point of view. They are local people who may just leave us alone. Granted they should be working in the fields and not causing trouble. It is what it is."

"Master, maybe they have weapons."

"Maybe they don't," said Liu.

"Master, we are walking into a known danger? The farmer has already warned us about what lies ahead. Wouldn't it be more prudent for us to get the local magistrate first to help us with the situation, or to try to find another road?"

"We have the advantage. We already know something is going to happen so we can prepare for it. A good martial artist is always alert to the possibility of an attack. You are training to become a martial artist. Of the Pa Kua Chang and Hsing-Yi Chuan I have taught you, what do you think are your strengths?"

"I like.."

"It is not what you like, but what you feel confident in using if the time comes for you to use it."

As they walked, Pei Ke started to think and compare the various martial art techniques he had learned from Liu.

"Pei Ke, it is too late," said Liu. "There is too much thinking on your part. If you need to think about it for so long, then you really don't have a good grasp of what you can and cannot do."

Pei Ke looked sheepishly at the ground. He felt embarrassed. Liu inwardly shook his head and chastised himself for not pushing Pei Ke harder. The boy needed to be a man and learn how to take care of himself. Learning new techniques is always good, and forms practice is good, but it is no substitute for actual contact with either an opponent or a sparring partner. Liu made a mental note to change Pei Ke's training.

As they walked down the road they could see the hillside closing in on both sides of the road. The rice paddies gave way to a bamboo forest which encroached closer and closer to the road until there was no separation between the bamboo and the road. The narrowing of the road and the overhanging bamboo forest gave the impression of entering into a long narrow cave. Pei Ke could reach out and touch the leaves.

Liu thought it was beautiful. He enjoyed the sight of bamboo, especially when there was a slight breeze. He always included bamboo in his paintings. He made a mental note to paint this very scene.

"Master, the bamboo forest is really dense. I feel as though we are being enclosed in a hollow tube. It makes me uncomfortable. Can we hurry?"

The sound of the rustling bamboo leaves reached them at the same time. The difference was that Liu was already reacting to the sound before Pei Ke was finished processing the implication of the sound. Liu didn't know what side the attack would come from, but he was ready for it. While Liu was moving, Pei Ke was frozen to one spot, unable to react to the situation.

Almost instantly, there were two men in front of them and two behind, all walking toward them. Liu thought they were about the same age as Pei Ke. One of the two in front stepped forward and with his left hand grabbed Liu's right wrist. Liu turned into the direction of the force. He could feel the strength of the man's grip. This one was strong for his age.

Liu hooked his right hand around the wrist of his opponent. He pulled the man's wrist slightly forward and then pushed back against the wrist, changing the angle of his opponent's elbow. As he turned more into the attack, Liu's left arm slid up against the opponents elbow. The upward direction of Liu's arm completely twisted the opponent's body. With a continuous downward spiraling movement of Pa Kua Chang, the opponent landed hard on the ground, his head hitting against a large stone, knocking him unconscious. It was over in less than two seconds.

Liu instantly rose upward into the ready position of Pa Kua Chang and moved towards the man next to him. The second opponent punched directly towards Liu's face as Liu switched from Pa Kua Chang to Hsing-Yi Chuan. The breaking of bones was swift and somewhat cruel. The opponent's right arm dropped limp and the man crumbled to the ground screaming in agony.

It had only been ten seconds and Pei Ke still stood, stunned. So did the other boys.

Finally snapping out of their inaction, they both charged. As fast as they moved, Liu moved faster, closing the distance so quickly that the two boys had no time to react. Before they could do anything, Liu used Pi Chuan and Bung Chuan movements from Hsing-Yi Chuan. The attackers fell with a broken nose and a cracked rib. The whole fight was over in less than twenty seconds.

Liu turned quickly and moved swiftly in his Pa Kua Chang ready position to thwart any other attack. As he surveyed the situation, he saw the four men down on the ground and Pei Ke standing looking around. He had not moved one inch.

"Master, do you need any help?"

"Pei Ke, it is all over! What help can you possibly give me?"

Pei Ke looked at Liu and felt embarrassed at what had happened. He was studying martial arts from a great master and when the time came for him to show what he had learned, he had completely frozen.

Liu walked over to the man with the broken nose, grabbed him by the collar, and yanked him to his feet. He was about Pei Ke's height and weight. The man immediately started swinging at Liu with his right hand. Liu immediately grabbed the arm and applied a Chin Na technique to the man's arm. Pain immediately shot up the man's arm.

"Pei Ke, I want you to stand two feet in front of this man."

"Master, he…"

"Don't ask questions. Do as I tell you to do."

Pei Ke could sense the change in Liu's voice as he stood directly in front of the man with the broken nose. Liu leaned close to the man's ear and whispered to him so Pei Ke could not hear.

Pei Ke could see the fear in the man's eyes and wondered what Liu was telling the man.

Liu continued whispering to the man. Liu adjusted his hold on the man's collar.

Again, he whispered to the man, "I do not know who you are or what you want from us, but if you do not follow my exact instructions you are going to die instantly. Now punch towards my student as hard as you can."

The man started to turn towards Liu and Liu grabbed the opponent's throat and squeezed. A gurgling sound came from the man as fear rose to overwhelm his body. Liu grasped harder on his collar to lift him and steady his footing.

Whispering one more time Liu said, "You are going to die now if you do not do as I ask. I am going to relax my grip on your throat and as soon as I do, punch towards my student."

Liu calculated the distance between the man he was holding and Pei Ke. He quickly released the grip on the man's throat. The man punched towards Pei Ke as fast as he could.

Pei Ke was startled when the punch came. The fist stopped one inch from Pei Ke's chest.

"Pei Ke!" shouted Liu. "Defend yourself."

"Master, what.."

"Quiet. Do not say another word."

Pei Ke had never heard Liu speak with such anger and forcefulness.

"Pei Ke, he is going to punch and I want you to defend against the attack. Do you understand?"

"Yes, Master."

"Punch," shouted Liu.

Pei Ke did nothing as fear rose upwards and spread throughout his body.

"Punch," shouted Liu once again.

This time Pei Ke moved to intercept the punch.

"Punch left, punch right, punch left."

Liu continued to yell out the commands and Pei Ke reacted to the punches. Liu leaned towards the man's ear and said, "Punch faster."

The man looked frantically at him as Liu subtly nudged him two inches closer. The man could not understand what was happening.

"Punch left, punch right," yelled Liu.

Pei Ke managed to just neutralize the first punch but was not able to do so with the second, which landed with a loud thud. Pei Ke looked startled as he fell backwards to the ground.

"Get up," shouted Liu. "Do it again."

Pei Ke got back into his previous position, and the punches started to fly. Some made their mark and others were blocked.

"Faster," yelled Liu.

Liu could tell after a minute that both of them were getting tired.

"Again!" shouted Liu.

Pei Ke was doing his best to keep up with the punches, but they were just too much for him. Liu sensed both were at the point of exhaustion.

"Stop," said Liu.

Liu turned to the man who had been throwing the punches. He looked exhausted.

"Gather up your friends and leave here immediately. If I ever see you again, I won't be so pleasant."

Liu and Pei Ke watched as the four men hobbled off down the road. When the men were fifty feet away, Liu turned towards Pei Ke and punched him. The blow caught Pei Ke in the abdomen and he crumbled to the ground.

"Pei Ke you must always be on guard. You never know when you will need to rely on your skills. Get up."

Pei Ke sensed the anger and frustration in Liu's voice, and he gingerly stood up and faced Liu.

"Don't you ever leave me to fight alone when you are able to help. Do you understand?"

"Yes, Master. I was..."

"Stop. Not another word. Let's continue on our journey."

Liu started walking and Pei Ke followed alongside of him. Both men were deep in thought. Pei Ke was trying to assimilate what had happened. He had never been hit like that before. His arms and chest were sore and were starting to feel bruised. He felt lucky. The man who had attacked him had been strong, but nowhere as strong as Liu. He knew Liu had held back with his punch and he shuddered to think what a full-blown attack from Liu would feel like. He thought of what Liu had told him. He was ashamed that Liu had chastised him for his inaction. He vowed to never let it happen again.

As they walked, Liu hoped the altercation on the road was a lesson for Pei Ke. The boy needed to be shocked into the reality that training in martial arts is a serious undertaking and not a game to be played at one's whim. He had been hard on Pei Ke, but the boy needed to learn and this was as good an opportunity as he could have. Pei Ke hadn't been hurt, beyond his pride, and hopefully he had made a resolution to not have this happen again.

From now on there would be more intense physical conditioning to teach Pei Ke how to take the punishment of getting hit. The boy had fallen down and bruised far too easily.

He looked at Pei Ke, who was showing alternating expressions of shame and determination, and nodded. Yes, it was definitely time to toughen Pei Ke up.

# CHAPTER NINE

On the fourth day, Liu and Pei Ke were traveling along a deserted stretch of road. They had not seen anyone or anything for several hours.

"Master, do you remember when we stayed at the inn and you treated Mrs. Wang?"

"Yes. It seems so long ago. Much has happened since we were there."

Liu thought of his family and those who had recently been brutally murdered by Chen Su and his son. Of course, Chen Chang had escaped and, as Liu had already so violently discovered, was still causing trouble. According to Hua Yee, there was another member of the gang and presumably, he had escaped as well. It was not difficult to believe that he had met up again with Chen Chang.

Liu remembered what the bounty hunter he had killed had said about the danger on the road, so he was on guard at all times, always prepared. An attack could come at any time. He needed to continue to train Pei Ke in the fundamentals of Chinese martial arts. As it stood now, he was still a liability in any altercation. Liu would have to keep protecting Pei Ke as well as defending himself.

"Master, I have a question."

"What is your question? Does it deal with martial arts or with acupuncture?"

"Acupuncture."

"Go ahead."

"Are there different types of headaches or migraines?"

"Why all of a sudden do you have this question?"

"I have been thinking about it for some time. I have been thinking about how you treated Mrs. Wang."

"Some doctors try to treat all headaches or migraines the same way. In ancient China, however, doctors identified as many as twenty-one different reasons for a person to have this particular condition."

"You mean a migraine can be treated in twenty-one different ways?"

"Yes, but let's not get fixated on the number twenty-one. Let's just say there are many reasons, and the astute doctor must determine which reason is causing the migraine for that particular patient. You can have numerous patients at the same time, each complaining of a migraine and each will have a different diagnosis and treatment. Do you understand?"

"Yes, Master. If there are different diagnoses, then there should be different prescriptions for both acupuncture treatments and herbal formulas to address each type of headache."

"Very good."

"Master, you've explained Liver Fire Rising before and how to differentiate it from Liver Blood Deficiency. What are some of the other reasons for migraines?"

"Not all doctors will agree with my answer, but migraines can be separated into two broad categories: interior and exterior.

"Interior migraines can be further divided into categories of excess and deficiency. In other words, there is either too much energy or not enough energy causing the migraine. Have I lost you yet?"

"No, Master. I understand. From what you've told me in the past; if there is an excess I don't want to increase the energy, and if there is a deficiency I don't want to deplete the energy."

"Yes. You are correct."

Pei Ke nodded proudly. He felt comfortable settling back into this master-student relationship. There was a lot to learn but he was determined to grasp it.

"Pei Ke, I have had you feel pulses. What would you expect to feel with a migraine patient who had an excess condition?"

Pei Ke thought for a moment.

"Master, if the patient had an excess condition and a migraine, I would expect the pulse to be strong."

"What if the pulse was weak?"

"Then I would expect the migraine was a deficiency condition."

"Good."

Pei Ke puffed up again, glad that he'd answered the question correctly.

"Pei Ke. In the interior excess category of migraines we can further isolate the cause. There would be liver energy problems such as Liver Yang Rising, Liver Fire Rising, Liver Wind, and Liver Qi Stagnation.

"There can also be elements causing the problem, such as wind, cold, dampness, and heat. Complicating it further, the pain could be caused by an injury of some sort. Sometimes this is classified as Blood Stasis. There could also be a combination of factors causing the problem. This is where the experience of the doctor, along with his training and clinical experience, help immensely."

"Master, is there one single factor differentiating one migraine from another?"

As soon as he'd asked the question he knew it was the wrong thing to ask.

With a barely audible sigh Liu turned to Pei Ke and said, "It is best to take all the signs and symptoms into consideration before making a diagnosis. For example, if the patient is female, I might suspect there is a hormonal connection to the migraine. If the migraine is on top of the head close to Bai Hui, point I might suspect there is a kidney energy connection. If the migraine is on the side of the head, there might be a large intestine or gall bladder energy problem. If the migraine is at the base of the neck, I might suspect a bladder or gall bladder connection. If the migraine is on the forehead it might lead me to question the patient about possible stomach or bladder problems. So once again it is a compilation of signs and symptoms leading us to a diagnosis.

"Let's take Liver Fire Rising, since you are familiar with the diagnosis. With Liver Fire Rising, I would expect to see the following: severe and intense throbbing in the head; dizziness and or vertigo; nausea and or vomiting; deafness and or tinnitus; red painful eyes; dry throat with thirst and a bitter taste in the mouth; constipation; and irritability and insomnia."

"Master, would you see all these symptoms?"

"Probably not, but you would see enough of them to lead you to a conclusion. Of course, you will need to take into consideration that a particular symptom might have more than one cause. As an example, if someone had nausea and vomiting there could be a wide range of diagnoses for that problem. Of course, you would do a tongue diagnosis and pulse diagnosis to help with your determination of the exact nature of the problem."

"Master, what would I expect with a tongue and or pulse diagnosis with Liver Fire Rising?"

"That is enough discussion for now on this excess condition. I could go on for hours on just this one topic. The other aspect of an interior problem is a deficiency. The deficiencies are usually, but not always, related to kidney, blood, and Qi. You need to be able to differentiate each one of them. As you can see, there are many more reasons why a migraine would be caused by an excess condition rather than a deficiency condition."

"Is this true in all situations or just with migraines?"

"Each health problem will have its own grouping of either excess or deficiency or both. Experience and study will help you to understand this more. All of the possibilities, causes, and symptoms we have been discussing are due to an interior problem. As I said before, there are also exterior problems causing migraines."

Pei Ke listened and wondered how he was ever going to remember all this material. Liu continued.

"Exterior conditions are caused by wind characteristics coupled with cold, heat, or dampness."

"Master, could you give me an example?"

"Yes." He thought for a moment trying to give Pei Ke a good example.

"I will give you a good example of a wind cold problem. On a cold winter day, you exercise quite strenuously, to the point that you are perspiring profusely. You take off your hat and coat and the cold wind blows on your body, especially your head and neck. The next day you have a headache, stiff neck, runny nose, and cough, and you are sneezing. You have just acquired the exterior problem of Wind Cold giving you a headache.

"Many doctors might suggest you are sick for another reason, but the symptoms are clear in this case."

"Master, how would you treat this Wind Cold problem?"

"Acupuncture and herbal formulas can relive the problem quickly. The patient should see some relief on the first visit to the Traditional Chinese Medicine doctor."

"Master, I would assume the number of acupuncture points would be based on the pulses."

"Yes, it would be based on the pulses and the imbalance of energy. However, from my experience, Feng Chi acupuncture point is very effective for this situation. Of course, I would use other points as well."

"What other uses would you have for this point?"

"Well, I find it effective for many wind problems, stiff neck and eye sight problems. That is enough information for now. Think about what I have taught you for awhile."

Pei Ke thought for a moment, trying to absorb the information. He needed many drawers in his head, like the drawers at the herbalist, to file all the information he was learning. He probably needed two sets of drawers. One set of drawers for the Traditional Chinese Medicine and another set for the martial arts he was learning. Hopefully, he would be able to remember it all when the time came for him to use it. Would there be enough space to add a few more drawers for painting, calligraphy, herbal medicine, feng shui, poetry, and all the other things Liu was going to teach him?

It suddenly dawned on him he had only known Liu for a couple of years. Why had Liu chosen him to receive part of the Liu fortune? There must be others he knew just as well if not better, like Uncle Wu or even Wei Ken De, who had been one of his senior students. And there was Tsao and Huo, who had both studied from Liu for much longer than he. There must be a reason he had been chosen. Maybe it was a plan of Liu's that included him. He realized that he had made the right decision when he had departed the temple instead of taking the treasure. Maybe it was a test, and there wasn't any treasure at all. Maybe Liu just wanted to see what he was going to do. Pei Ke continued walking along the road with Liu, totally oblivious to his surroundings.

# CHAPTER TEN

On the sixth day, Liu woke up as usual. He had trained himself since childhood to wake up before sunrise. Today was no different. He walked over to where Pei Ke was sleeping and nudged him with his foot.

"Pei Ke, it is time to get up. We have a long way to travel today and I want to get started early."

Pei Ke rolled over and mumbled something. For most of the night, Pei Ke had dreamt about some of his experiences since he and Liu had begun their initial trip to Liu's ancestral village. First he'd dreamt of the river crossing and the fight Liu had had in the small boat as they'd crossed from one side of the river to the other. Then he'd dreamt of his part in the death of the man outside Chen Su's camp.

Liu nudged Pei Ke once again. Pei Ke could feel the cold floor. As he turned, he felt the ache in his muscles.

They had found shelter for the night with a farmer who let them sleep in an attached room to the house. They didn't have entry to the house, and the only warmth came from a makeshift hole in the wall that let in some heat. They both had slept on the cold stone floor with a light blanket provided by the farmer.

"Master, I ache all over."

"The coldness of the floor has entered into your body. You need exercise to rid your body of this evil coldness. If you do not exercise, then some part of the coldness may remain and adversely affect you later."

Pei Ke remembered what Liu had told him about external factors entering the body and causing physical problems. Reluctantly, he rose and followed Liu in their morning exercise ritual.

The farmer was kind enough to provide them with some rice and vegetables for breakfast. After eating, they embarked once more on their journey toward Beijing. At first, in the early morning with little or no light, they walked in silence, but after they had walked for a while and the sun had started to warm their bodies, Pei Ke turned to Liu.

"Master, I remember our discussion about the herb Tang Kuei and its value to women with hormonal issues. What other herbs should I be familiar with?"

"Tang Kuei is probably the most important herb for women. It helps to relieve many of the symptoms women experience not only in their developmental and mothering years but also in later life when their menses cease. Do you remember what I told you before about it?"

"Yes, Master. I remember everything you taught me."

"It is important that you do not forget this information. What I have taught you will be useful when you have a need to treat women.

"The next herb you should remember is Ren Shen. It is the root of the plant we are most interested in. It is one of those primary herbs in Chinese medicine that has many therapeutic qualities. Thus, it is used quite often in many diverse formulas.

"Its name is characteristic of how it can look. Often it will look like the torso of a man with two legs. Thus, it's characteristic name of 'man root'. It was first mentioned in the Divine Husbandman's Classic of the Materia Medica, authored by Shen Nung. When I was in Shanghai, I met a western-trained doctor who knew of it in the west. It was used by some of the native Indians. In the west it is called ginseng.

"It has many varieties. One variety is red Ren Shen which comes from Korea. It has slightly different properties than the Chinese variety and is a little more potent. Even here in China there are slightly different varieties. Wild Ren Shen is found in many different areas of this vast land. Those who search for it usually find it in remote regions, in a wooded, shaded mountainous environment with well-drained loose soil.

"It has a slightly sweet and bitter taste and has a slight warming effect on the body. It has a direct tonification effect on the lung and spleen meridians. As such, it is used in treating lung problems such as shortness of breath. Since it is a tonifying herb, it can be used in cases where there is depleted Qi. It is almost always used in combination with one or more other herbs depending on the differential diagnosis. It can be used in formulas treating infertility and impotency. Of course, the composition of the formula, dosage, and the amount of Ren Shen will vary based on the diagnostic pattern."

"Master, should we eat ginseng by itself?"

"There may be some instance where you can drink ginseng brew by itself, but it is better to boil it with other herbs and then drink the concoction. You need to be careful with Ren Shen, just like the other Chinese herbs. There are, for example, contraindications and toxicity levels. Patients with high blood pressure and excess heat conditions should not take too much of it."

He looked at Pei Ke.

"Can you remember all this?"

"Yes, Master. Actually, as I said before, the more you teach me, the easier it is for me to learn. I just need to memorize the new names."

"Are you ready to learn about another herb?"

"Of course," said Pei Ke.

"The next herb is Ma Huang."

"Master, this was the herb you gave to the monk at the temple just before we went to your brother's home, wasn't it?"

"Yes. Your memory is good. The herb is used quite often for lung problems."

Liu went on to describe the herb, where it was primarily grown, and its therapeutic properties. Then he taught Pei Ke about three other herbs as they continued their journey eastward.

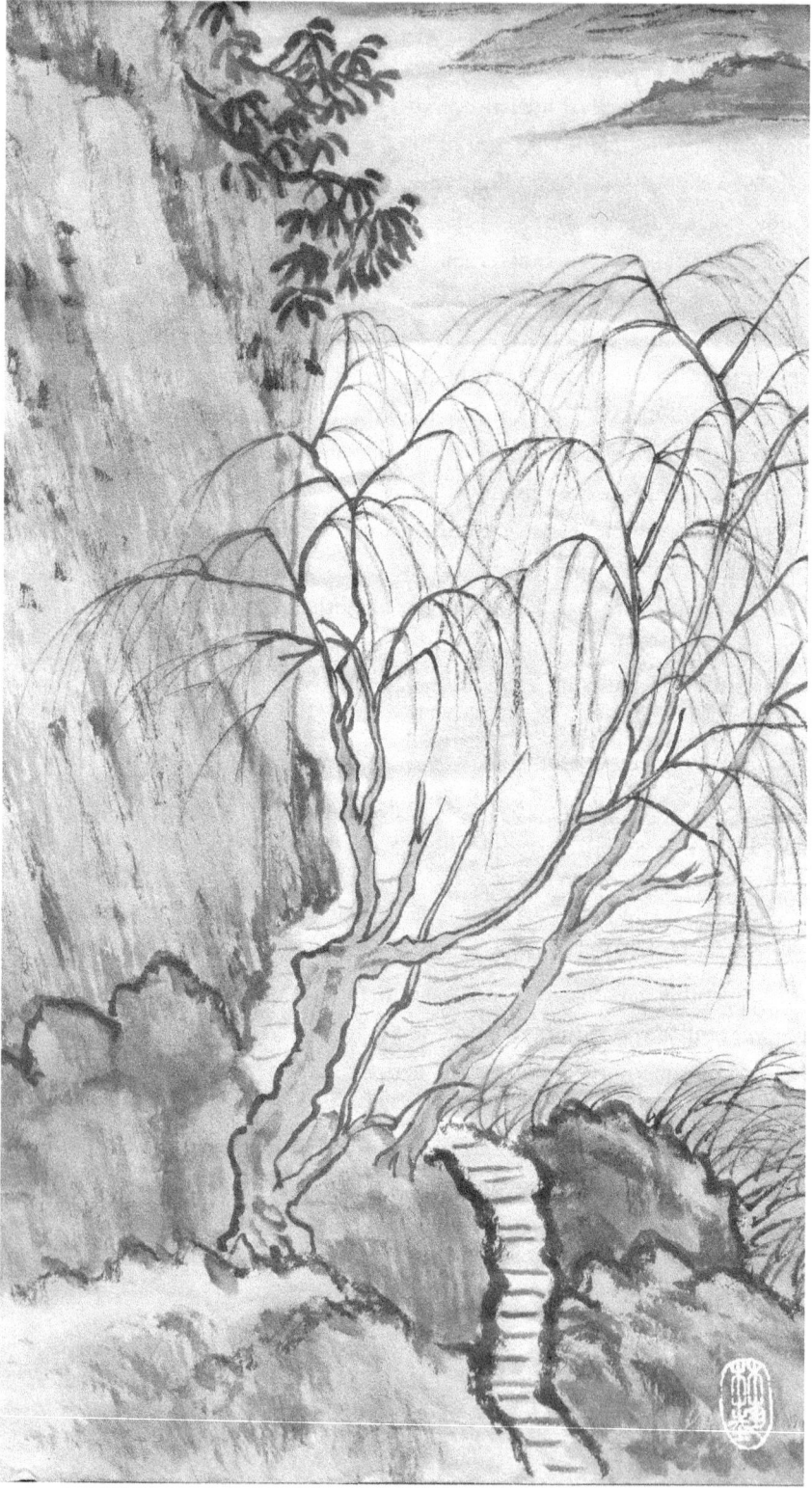

# CHAPTER ELEVEN

On the seventh, day they came to the outskirts of what appeared to be a small village. It was on the banks of a wide, slow-moving river, typical of many rivers in that region of China. As Pei Ke and Liu looked down the river, they saw numerous boats bobbing on the water. They briefly watched as the village men tended to their fishing nets.

It was idyllic, with bamboo trees spreading out from the river to meet lush green fields. The village and its surroundings were situated in such a way that the whole scene appeared to be protected by an invisible force.

As they entered the village, they realized the scene had been deceptive. For one thing, the village was not as small as it appeared. Children played in the streets and villagers went about their daily activities.

"Master, this village looks quite nice. In fact, it is probably the cleanest and nicest place I've seen in a long time."

"You are right; it does look nice. It is laid out appropriately and someone seems to have spent a considerable amount of time convincing the local populace to keep the place neat and tidy."

As they walked towards the center of the village, an elderly man who was tall and lanky approached them. His stature and clothes set him apart from the others, giving the impression that he was someone who held a position of importance or authority.

"How are you?" he said as he approached. "I see you are strangers to this village. I am the local magistrate, and I like to know who is visiting us."

"My name is Liu Bin, and this is Pei Ke. We are traveling to Beijing, but it is getting late in the day. Is there a temple we can visit and stay for the night and maybe have a meal?"

"Are you a monk? Your clothes certainly suggest an affiliation with some religious sect."

"I am not a monk, but I do live with them. I follow my own religious beliefs, but I am conversant with medicine and I have often been able to help the monks in exchange for lodging and food for the evening. Is there a temple in the area?"

"What kinds of problems can you help with?"

"Is there a doctor in this village?"

"There was, but he passed away last year. Now the nearest doctor is over a day's journey and many can't make the trip, especially if they are critically ill."

"I have experience in treating a wide range of health issues. Is there someone in the village who needs help?"

"Yes, my neighbor is seriously ill. She has been sick for a few days. We are keeping her comfortable, but we don't know what to do for her. She is running a fever along with some other symptoms. And to answer your question, there is no temple here. But if you need a place to stay for the night, we can make arrangements with someone in the village. May I presume your companion is studying medicine with you?"

"Yes, he is studying with me. We appreciate any accommodations you might have. Who is this person you want me to see?"

The man blushed and bowed slightly.

"If you don't mind, I must talk with her first and get her permission."

"I understand."

"There is a large tree in the center of the village." The man pointed in the direction of the tree. "Why don't you and your student wait next to the tree, and I will let the family know."

Liu and Pei Ke walked towards the center of the village as the elderly gentleman went off towards the southern edge of the village.

The tree was exactly where it was supposed to be. In fact, it couldn't be missed, as it was huge and quite old. There were worn but sturdy wooden benches by the tree and Liu and Pei Ke were just getting comfortable when the man returned.

"She will see you," he said with relief. "Her condition has not deteriorated, as far as I can tell, but it is not getting any better either."

Liu and Pei Ke walked in silence as they followed the man to the southern part of the village. They turned at one corner, then another. The area was amazingly clean without any writings or posters hanging from the walls or poles. Pei Ke was impressed by the pride the people took in their village.

Finally, they stopped at a red double door, and the magistrate knocked. Soon a tall, muscular man opened the door. Liu knew immediately that the man knew some form of martial arts. He couldn't have explained to Pei Ke how he knew, but he knew. Sometimes he could tell by the way a person moved or the way they walked. But in this case, he wasn't entirely sure how he knew. He just did.

Liu also sensed that the man was reading him in a similar way. They stared at each other for a few seconds, then the magistrate explained why they were there, unaware of what had passed.

Almost reluctantly, they were escorted into a courtyard. As they walked into the area, Pei Ke saw that several of the trees had bark that was damaged or scraped off.

Liu noticed this as well, and though he understood its significance, Pei Ke did not. It confirmed Liu's instinct, however, as the mangled trees were definite proof that someone here was practicing martial arts and they had a significant degree of expertise. It was not easy to inflict that type of damage to a tree without a certain amount of skill to prevent oneself from getting hurt.

From the location of the damage, Liu knew the scarring was due to high kicks, which meant this practitioner was familiar with one or more of the external martial arts. Internal martial arts did not emphasize high kicks.

Liu and Pei Ke were shown into a modest looking home. There were the customary statues and incense sticks burning on a miniature altar. Anyone visiting would think it was just an ordinary house with all the appropriate trimmings.

They were directed to sit and the magistrate and the man who'd met them at the door disappeared. Pei Ke turned to Liu and was about to ask a question, but Liu put his finger to his lips.

After a few minutes, the door opened slowly and a short, robust man entered the room and quickly walked over to Liu. As he approached, Liu stood up and Pei Ke was struck by how much taller Liu was.

"Welcome to my home. My name is Shen Yang. I understand that you are a doctor. Is that correct?"

Liu nodded.

"My name is Liu Bin. I have studied medicine for most of my life. I live with a group of monks in an area south of here, about three weeks journey by foot. This is Pei Ke, who is one of my students. We are on our way to Beijing to visit some of my friends.

"I understand that there is someone here who may need help. I would like to exchange my services for lodging and food for the night."

"It is true that my wife has not been feeling well for the last few days. But we do not know you. How can we know that you are who you say you are, and that you can do what you say you can do?"

"I do not know how to reassure you but to invite you to watch and ask me questions."

For the next fifteen or twenty minutes, Liu and Shen Yang talked about medicine and other topics. Pei Ke found the conversation very enlightening. Shen Yang seemed to know a little about medicine and his questions were direct and to the point. Liu answered confidently and patiently. Toward the end of the conversation, Liu began to ask some questions of his own.

"Tell me about your wife. What is wrong with her?"

"She has a bad sore throat with recurring chills for the last few days," Shen Yang said. "It came on very quickly, and I suggested she stay indoors. Do you think you can help her?"

"Is there an herbalist in this village?"

"No, we don't have an herbalist. There was a doctor who lived here and took care of the villagers, but he died last year. He had a small supply of herbs and would dispense them to the villagers as needed, but those are gone now too. Ever since he died, we've been looking for a new doctor to come and join our community. We don't have a lot of money but as a community we express appreciation by contributing as much as possible to support the doctor."

He sighed and shook his head. Then he looked back at Liu.

"If you'll follow me, I will take you to my wife."

After introductions were made, Liu turned to Pei Ke.

"Watch and listen," he said.

Liu felt the woman's pulses. He started out on the right side and then felt the pulses on the left wrist. Pei Ke watched intently remembering how Liu had taught him to feel the radial artery on the wrist, the three locations on each wrist, and the two depths of readings. Liu spent a few minutes with each wrist. He knew from years of experience that this process was one of the determining factors in a diagnosis, and he didn't want to hurry the process. He wanted to be accurate.

"Pei Ke I want you to feel her pulses."

Liu watched intently as Pei Ke sat down next to the woman. Mentally, Pei Ke went through a checklist he had put together. He knew this day would come and that Liu would be scrutinizing his every move.

"Pei Ke, take your time. There is no hurry here."

The woman looked at Liu, and he gave her a reassuring smile. She gave a half-hearted smile in return, and looked back at Pei Ke, wondering what he was going to do.

"Mrs. Yang, what are your symptoms?" asked Liu.

"My biggest complaint is my sore throat," she said. "It started a couple of days ago and is not getting any better. I also have intermittent chills and fever and a headache that is all over but worse on the side of my head. But my throat is the real issue. It hurts from top to bottom."

Mrs. Yang pointed to the area where she had the sore throat.

"Is it sore on both sides of your throat, or just where you pointed?" asked Liu.

"In the same area on both sides."

"Pei Ke, what have you found?"

"Master, she has a rapid pulse. The pulse is superficial rather than deep."

"Look at her tongue and tell me what you find."

Mrs. Yang stuck out her tongue. Pei Ke and Liu both looked.

"What do you see?"

"Master, her tongue is slightly red and there is a thin yellow coating on the surface."

"Pei Ke, what would you expect with a red tongue and a yellow coating?"

"Both of these indicate there is heat in her body."

"You are correct."

"Master, what does that mean?" asked Mrs. Yang.

"It means there is heat in your body, and it is causing you to have a sore throat. The Lung Meridian runs from your chest to your thumb. There is an internal pathway that communicates with the throat. There are usually two possible reasons for a sore throat, either an excess or a deficiency. In your case I suspect you have an excess of heat. The other possibility is a Yin deficiency. But with a Yin deficiency, the sore throat usually comes on gradually. In many cases, when a Yin deficiency causes a sore throat, the tongue is red but there is an absence of yellow coating on the tongue. You have a distinct yellow coating. In both cases, the pulse would be rapid, but in a Yin deficiency it would be thready, whereas yours is superficial."

"So is it serious?" asked Mrs. Yang.

"It is not serious and you should see some results quickly. Is it alright for me to treat you with acupuncture?"

"Yes, of course," said Mrs. Yang.

"Pei Ke, the treatment I am going to do is a little different from what you have seen before. I need to get some of the heat out of her lungs, so I am going to use the Shao Shang acupuncture point. Watch what I am doing so you can do it when you see someone with similar conditions."

Liu did the treatment as Pei Ke watched. As the woman was resting, Pei Ke asked questions and Liu answered them. Pei Ke was especially inquisitive about the unique technique Liu used on the Shao Shang acupuncture point.

"Master, do you use that technique whenever there is heat in the body?"

"There are different ways to get rid of heat in the body and in the meridians. In this case, the treatment was appropriate for her. Gradually you will learn the different conditions and when and what is appropriate."

That night they were invited to stay in the village and were given food and a place to stay.

# CHAPTER TWELVE

On the ninth day, they rose just before sunrise. Even so, the monks who had been generous enough to allow them to stay the night were already up when Liu and Pei Ke arose. They had been fortunate the night before to find a small Buddhist temple on the outskirts of a small village. It was picturesque, built on a large hill overlooking the surrounding community.

The road leading up to the temple reminded Pei Ke of a large undulating snake. The temple itself was much like the other temples they had visited during their journeys. There were the various statues of the deities and of course there was the ever present statue of Kuan Yin. For a small community it had a rather large area for worship. The colors of red and gold were present as he would have anticipated.

In the morning Liu invited the monks to join him and Pei Ke in their morning practice of his specialized style of Qi Gong. Afterward the monks had many questions. They crowded around Liu and Pei Ke. Pei Ke listened carefully to the questions and quickly realized that, while the monks regularly did their own form of Qi Gong, their understanding of the importance of structural alignment was lacking and very superficial. While the monks watched, Liu demonstrated a few of the more critical concepts of body alignment.

After the practice, Liu and Pei Ke joined the monks for a breakfast of soy bean milk and an assortment of vegetables and flour buns.

Pei Ke had had this type of bun before when he had lived with his parents. It had been a delicacy that he'd looked forward to once a week. The difference between the buns the monks ate and his parent's buns were the content. The buns his parents purchased at the market were filled with pork and a special plum sauce. He could see them now and that succulent taste flooded his mind.

These buns that the monks ate, which looked almost the same, had very thin clear rice noodles inside with a variety of chopped vegetables and lots of onions. They were good. In fact, they were really good, especially since he was hungry this morning, but they did not substitute for what he really was craving.

After breakfast Liu and Pei Ke said goodbye to the monks and continued their easterly journey towards Beijing. Pei Ke was deep in thought and was about to ask Liu a question when Liu spoke.

"Pei Ke, what do you think causes disease?"

"Master the cause of disease is an imbalance in the Qi flowing through our bodies."

"No. That is the result of the disease process. I asked you the cause of disease. We have discussed this before, but not in great detail. It is important for you to know the causative factors that lead to the disease process.

"These are two separate things and you need to distinguish them in your mind. The first is the causative factor and the second is the disease process where the body changes due to the causative factors. Do you understand the difference?"

"I think so," said Pei Ke.

"Basically, what is the cause and what is the result? It is important to know the general factors of both of these. The body should be in a balanced state and that balanced state is what each of us strives for in our life. However, there are constant impingements on our bodies, affecting that balanced condition. Each of us has the ability to adjust to the impingements to one degree or another, but when we can't make the adjustment ourselves, then the disease process sets in. This is where doctors come in to help the body. The doctor helps put you back together when you become unbalanced and cannot return to the balanced condition on your own.

"Our ancestors discovered numerous factors causing disease. These include weather-related conditions, emotions, diet, strain, physical exercise, bodily injuries, animal bites, blood issues, and bodily fluids. I have touched on some of this in our previous discussion, but I am going to elaborate on them now. Pay attention and make sure you understand what I am telling you.

"There are six external weather-related causative factors affecting the human body. At first, there is a tendency to dismiss the weather as a causative factor, but when you understand the relationships you will be able to understand what is happening in the human body. Quite often, the change of the seasons will affect the human body. This is quite prevalent when there is a change from autumn to winter. I am sure you've heard people complain of sickness when there are sudden changes from warm weather to cold weather and back again."

"Master, I remember my mother telling me to be careful when the weather changes so I don't catch a cold or get the flu. She also went to the herbalist four times a year to get herbs to help all of us make the transition from one season to another."

"Your mother was very wise. I am sure what she did helped you to stay healthy throughout the year. So you understand from your personal experience that there are weather related factors influencing our bodies.

"The first of these factors I want you to understand is the factor of wind. Wind can come at any time of the year, but it is the most influential in our bodies when it comes during the change of the season. The ancients discovered that wind will attack or invade the body after sweating or while one is sleeping. Therefore, it is important when sleeping to have a cover or blanket over you to protect yourself.

"I have treated patients who would leave a window open so the air could circulate through their bedroom. The air from the outside would blow across their bodies and quite often they would wake up in the morning not feeling well. They would attribute their ailment to restless sleep when, in truth, it was the wind causing the problem. Many times we refer to the wind as 'Evil Wind' since it can affect us so strongly and is a leading cause of many diseases. The ancients also realized that wind can combine with other factors such as cold and dampness to invade the body."

"Master, of course the air is cold during winter, but it's much colder when the wind is blowing. It feels like the cold can enter the body faster when there's wind than when there's no wind."

"Yes, the wind does accentuate the essence of coldness. Now, do you think the wind is a Yang factor or a Yin factor?"

Pei Ke thought for a moment. He knew that Yang factors were external and Yin factors were internal. He also knew anything Yang had a tendency to move while those things Yin had a tendency to be still.

"Master, I think wind has the characteristics of being Yang."

"Yes, you are correct," said Liu. "Now is it upward or downward?"

Pei Ke thought once again. He remembered Liu telling him Yin was inside and downward so wind must be upward.

"Master, wind is upward and outward. Is that correct?"

"Yes," said Liu. "Thus it affects the upper part of the body causing headaches, and problems related to the eyes, nose, throat, and ears.

"Since wind never blows in one steady stream, but in gusts, one characteristic of wind is its ability to travel. One of the factors of changing pain problems is due in part to the wind in the body traveling from one place to another. It is also believed that wind may be the cause of some of our skin problems such as itching and skin eruptions that come and go on different parts of our body."

"Master, my sister had an outbreak of raised, red wheals on her body. They came and went and she said they itched. I remember seeing her in the morning with the wheals on one part of her arm and in the evening on another part of her arm. Is this the kind of thing you're talking about?"

"It could be. It could also be something else, but I would definitely consider wind as a potential cause.

"The ancients also discovered that wind can cause such problems as dizziness, facial paralysis, eye watering, and headaches. I have treated many patients complaining of headaches when the wind blows especially during the change of seasons."

"Master, since the wind affects the body so adversely it must be important to avoid the effects of the wind."

"Yes, this is especially important when the pores are open due to exercise or while sleeping. When I was in Beijing, a very wealthy man came to see me about pain is his neck. When I questioned him about his habits, he indicated he always slept with the window open. He liked the feeling of wind blowing across his body. I explained to him the adverse effects of his actions. I treated him with acupuncture and sent him home. A few days later he came to see me and thanked me for helping him. My advice on closing the window made all the difference in his pain."

"Master, if wind is such a problem, then there must be a way in Traditional Chinese Medicine to treat this problem."

"Yes," said Liu. "There is more than one way to treat it. The doctor can use acupuncture, herbs, Tui Na, or a combination of the these. As I mentioned to you before, one of the major acupuncture points is Feng Chi, which literally means 'pond of wind.' It is believed that this is one of the points where the wind collects in the body. Inserting a needle into this point releases the collection of wind. I use this point anytime someone has cold or flu-like symptoms. There is a special way to insert the needle into this point. If done wrong, it could do harm to the patient. I will show you the technique next time we need to use this point."

"Master, can you show me where the point is located?"

Liu pointed to the location of the point and helped Pei Ke locate it on his own body.

"Master, on which meridian is this point located?"

"It is located on the Gall Bladder Meridian."

"Can it be used to treat gall bladder problems?"

"In theory any point on a meridian can be used to treat its respective organ. However, generations of practitioners have found certain points to be more effective than others. And to answer your question, I would not use that point to treat gall bladder problems. I would probably use other points and combinations of points to treat gall bladder problems."

"Master, what else do I need to know about wind?"

"There is more for you to learn, but we've talked enough about wind for today. You should understand and remember each of these causes, so let's move on to the factor of cold and how it affects the body."

Pei Ke nodded. He trusted his master's method of teaching, but was always disappointed when Liu changed subjects just when they were getting interesting.

"Cold is more likely to affect the body in winter than any other season. It is a Yin factor and affects the warmth of the body. As it affects the body, the arms and legs become cold, the abdominal area may be cold, and the patient may experience loose bowels or diarrhea. As the body becomes cold, there may be tight tendons and muscles with the possibility of muscle injury with overexertion. Cold can combine with wind to cause headaches and stiff neck.

"Summer heat, on the other hand, is seen almost exclusively in the summer when the temperature is high. It is a Yang factor and is caused by excessive heat, such as you might find when working too long in the fields and being exposed to the sun. Since it is a Yang factor, like wind, it most often affects the upper part of the body giving rise to fever, dizziness, thirst, dry eyes, dry mouth, sunstroke, restlessness, sweating, and weakness. Summer heat can also be combined with wind, which brings the symptoms on more quickly and in a more exaggerated manner."

"Master, is this why some people feel lightheaded if the temperature is too hot?"

"Yes," said Liu. "There is also a classification of heat. There is a difference between Summer Heat and other heat. Summer heat is more intense and obviously is seen in the hottest part of the summer. Other heat symptoms can be seen other times of the year and their symptoms while similar are less intense.

"Now, the next factor is dampness. Dampness can be seen any time of the year, but its pathogenic nature is more predominant in the latter part of summer. It is a Yin factor. As you can imagine, dampness comes about by exposure to dampness or prolonged exposure to moisture. You often see it in people who work in rice paddies or people who are exposed to rain for extended periods of time. You would not expect to see a lot of this type of condition in the desert where there is little water.

"With dampness, you can expect to hear complaints of heaviness in the body, painful joints, arthritic pain in the joints, loose stools, undigested food in the stools, swelling and water retention, fullness in the chest, and fullness in the abdominal area causing lack of appetite. Since the spleen deals with dampness, we can choose points on the Spleen Meridian to effectively treat this problem."

"Master, are there points of the Spleen Meridian that you prefer to use?"

"The points San Yin Jiao and Yin Ling Quan are effective in treating dampness problems. Be careful not to use San Yin Jiao when a woman is pregnant. For women who have difficulty in going to full term in their pregnancy, it might cause fetal distress, and the mother could lose the baby."

Liu pointed to the two points on his own body and then watched as Pei Ke located them on his body.

"Good, you are getting better at locating points."

# CHAPTER THIRTEEN

On the tenth day, Liu and Pei Ke found themselves on a road running parallel to a medium-sized stream. They had walked for about a mile when Liu stopped and walked over to a large flat boulder situated between the road and the stream. He looked at the water for a while and motioned for Pei Ke to sit on the boulder with him.

The wind was cold as it blew out of the north. Pei Ke thought of the wind-cold discourse he recently had with Liu and sat to the right of Liu. Liu acted as a shield for the cold wind, which didn't seem to bother him in the least.

Pei Ke thought, *He must have a different type of blood inside of him to keep him warm. Or his years of Qi Gong and martial arts practice have conditioned him to ignore discomfort.*

Pei Ke was going to ask some questions, but Liu was staring thoughtfully at the stream and Pei Ke guessed he wouldn't answer any questions. They sat there for a long time absorbed in their own thoughts.

Pei Ke's thoughts again turned to the events of the last couple of months. He had experienced so much in such a short period of time. It was true what his parents told him about one's fortune. It could change in an instant; either for the better or for worse. For him, it had surely changed for the better.

He remembered the time he had first discovered Liu practicing. It had simply been chance that he'd chosen that morning to get up early and explore the mountain. If he hadn't he probably would never have met Liu and experienced all he had experienced. The gods were surely looking after him. He wondered what the gods had in store for him in the future. He hoped it included a continuation of his studies with Liu.

Pei Ke looked at Liu.

"Do you have a question?" asked Liu without looking over.

"Master, sometimes I am a little hesitant to ask questions. I know that my questions seem to come continuously as if they are coming from a list of things to ask you one after another. It is just that there is so much to ask you and the more that I learn from you the more that I realize what I don't know and the more questions I need to ask. Opening one door of knowledge leads to two doors which lead to three more doors."

"What is the question," asked Liu.

"Master, your training in martial arts includes Tai Chi Chuan, Pa Kua Chang, and Hsing-Yi Chuan. From what you have told me, this training has also included classical weapons. In Tai Chi Chuan the main weapon is a sword. Am I correct?"

"Yes, sword is the classical weapon in Tai Chi Chuan, but not the only weapon. There is also the broad sword and the long staff."

"What about the Hsing-Yi Chuan and Pa Kua Chang weapons?"

"I think it is strictly a preference, but in Hsing-Yi Chuan I prefer the broad sword because of its slicing capabilities. Of the weapons in Pa Kua Chang I prefer the Deer Horn Knives. In my opinion, the Deer Horn Knives are the most lethal and versatile weapons in existence."

"What makes them so unique?" asked Pei Ke. "I have never seen them, but I've seen a Tai Chi sword."

"The Deer Horn Knives look like two half moons hooked together. The weapon is held in the middle where the two moons cross."

He drew the shape of the knives on the palm of his hand.

"This is the basic shape of the Deer Horn Knife. Each surface is a cutting surface except for the handle. Most people who practice Pa Kua Chang are familiar with this shape. I prefer to use an enhanced set of Deer Horn Knives that are longer and have an extra curve used for hooking. In my opinion, however, the Deer Horn Knives are an advanced weapon. It would be better for the beginning student to learn the sword or broadsword. You should learn more about Pa Kua Chang and Hsing-Yi Chuan before you start learning weapons."

"Master, the only weapon I've seen looked like it was either a short knife or a sword. Since I've seen this weapon, will you tell me more? How do you use the Tai Chi sword?"

"Before I teach you how to use the sword, you need to know more about the sword itself. The history of the sword goes back many generations. There have been many famous sword makers and swordsmen.

"There are different sword forms and different emphasis on sword usage depending on who teaches the sword form. Even though there are different sword forms, the principles for all the sword forms should be similar. Basically, the sword is used for stabbing, cutting, slicing, and blocking.

"Do you remember what the Tai Chi sword looks like?"

"Yes, Master. There is the sword blade and the handle."

"Correct, but there is more than just a blade and a handle. The Tai Chi sword is composed of the tip, wide portion of the straight blade, cutting edge, hand guard, handle, and pommel.

"Each part has a function and you should know the functions of the sword to be able to defend yourself. In addition, there is the scabbard which holds the sword; it also has a function.

"The tip of the sword is used for penetrating the body with a thrust-like motion. This can be done with an upwards, downwards, or horizontal motion. The thrust can be to any part of the body, but is most often used when attacking the torso of the opponent. The tip is also used for a quick cut against the tendons of a joint, particularly the knee and the ankle. We choose these areas of the body because they are more stationery than the wrist and elbow which are in continuous motion.

"The blade and handle together make up the length of the sword. The length of the sword is different for each individual. There is more than one way to determine the optimum length of the sword. One way is to measure the distance from the top of the instep of the foot to the center of the umbilicus. This would be the total length of the sword including the handle. The grip part of the handle would be one and a half hand widths long.

"The sword itself is wider in the middle than at the cutting edge. This is true for the entire length of the sword except near the tip. When one blocks with the sword, especially against another edged blade, the sword metal has a tendency to break at the point of impact. It is more resilient and stronger at the widest area which is the middle of the blade. Thus, it is appropriate whenever possible to use the middle or center of the sword to block another edged weapon.

"The cutting edge of the sword is on both sides of the blade. This is in contrast to the broad sword which has a cutting edge only on one side. The function of the broad sword and the straight sword are different. I will explain the differences later when we discuss the broad sword.

"The cutting edge is used in either a slicing or a hacking movement or a combination of both. The movement of the sword can be horizontal, vertical, or sideways. Usually, it is done with the sword being pulled away from the opponent during the attack, but it is conceivable the sword could be used towards the opponent.

"The handle should be wide enough for a person to grasp the sword with one hand where the thumb crosses over the index and middle fingers.

"The pommel is at the base of the sword and gives balance to the sword. Because of its weight it can also be used to hit your opponent."

"Master, I didn't realize there was so much to learn about a sword. I assume there is significant information to learn about each weapon."

"Yes, each weapon, whether it is from the external martial arts or the internal martial arts has its own characteristics and principles of usage. When the principles are followed, along with an understanding of the weapon, then the person using the weapon can be a formidable opponent. It is the person who has only a cursory knowledge of the weapon who is dangerous. He is only dangerous to himself and those he thinks he is protecting. I want you to be good at weapons before you decide to carry one. Do you understand?"

"Yes, Master. I understand."

"Let me continue with what I was saying. The balance is an important aspect of any sword. If the weight is too far forward then the sword is top heavy and difficult to control. If the weight is too far back it is difficult to judge the location of the blade. Each sword should be tailor-made for the individual. When this is done and there is the correct balance point with the sword, then the swordsman can practice with the sword so the sword becomes an integral part and extension of his arm. When this takes place, the sword is an extension of the Qi of the body.

"An experienced swordsman can immediately tell if the sword in his hand is his sword. This is possible even if all physical aspects of the sword seem identical. The sword becomes part of the man, and the man becomes part of the sword. A good sword is worth a lot of money to an adept swordsman. He will do everything possible to keep his sword, and it is an honor for the sword to be passed down from father to son."

"Master, did your father have a favorite sword?"

"Yes, the weapons should have been at my ancestral home. But they were missing when we arrived there. I asked Mr. Wu if he knew where they were but he did not know. I assume they were stolen by those who killed my family. There were many weapons including swords, knives, broad swords, staffs, and other weapons. The sword and knife that I took from the hiding place as you know were given to Mr. Wu for safe keeping."

"When we started the journey to your parent's home, did you leave any weapons at the temple?"

"Is that important?"

"No, Master. I was just curious since you did not carry a sword and …"

Pei Ke stopped talking sensing Liu did not want to answer the question. They both were silent for awhile before Liu spoke. It was a strange moment. Over the months of his apprenticeship, Liu had avoided his questions for many reasons, but never because of some personal tragedy. Pei Ke looked down, embarrassed, but Liu saved him.

"I did not finish what I was telling you about the sword," said Liu. "The sword is held in the right hand. The left hand is used to hold the scabbard which can be used to block or deflect an attack. If you do not have a scabbard in the left hand then the index and middle fingers of that hand are held out together. The ring and little fingers curl into the center of the palm and are covered with the thumb. This gives the swordsman balance, as though he had two swords, one in each hand.

"There is actually a double sword and some individuals are very good with two swords. One sword is in each hand and they are used to block, slice, and stab—alternatively or together—keeping the opponent off balance."

"Master, do you know double Tai Chi sword?"

"Yes. I will teach you someday."

Pei Ke thought about all the weapons he was going to learn from Liu. Simply becoming proficient in a single weapon would take months, let alone learning all that Liu knew. Pei Ke mentally calculated that for him to learn everything Liu knew, it would take years. Maybe he could give up eating and sleeping, and then just maybe he could learn it all. Pei Ke wondered how Liu remembered it all.

# CHAPTER FOURTEEN

aster, we have been traveling for a long time. Initially, we traveled from the temple, where I first met you, to your ancestral home; and now from your ancestral home to Beijing. Since we started traveling months ago, numerous people have attacked you. When you defend yourself, it seems so effortless. On a few occasions, I've seen you touch certain parts of your opponent's body. Can you explain why you do that?"

"There are certain acupuncture points and Ahsi Points that are effective in self defense. I will teach you about them."

Pei Ke suddenly became very alert and Liu debated whether or not he should share this with his student. Most martial artists know specific points on the body that can be used in self defense, but there were very few martial artists who really knew how and when to use these and other points. The information was kept secret and only passed on to the most advanced inner door students. He looked at Pei Ke, and a voice deep inside of him suggested what he needed to do. He needed to give Pei Ke a small taste of what was to come.

"As you know, the energy in our body flows along the meridian system. Do you remember me telling you before about the energy being circular and that there is neither a beginning point nor an ending point? It is in continuous motion."

"Yes, Master. I remember. You told me to visualize the energy as a circular tube filled with energy. To keep the energy from becoming stagnant it flows along this tube."

"Good. The ancient Chinese discovered that as the energy flows, there are particular times of the day when the energy is at its maximum. This changes every two hours and corresponds to the organs of the body. We can assume the opposite side of the circle is where there is the least amount of energy.

"Do you remember what I told you about the liver? Between eleven in the evening and one in the morning, the energy of the Liver Meridian is at its maximum."

"Yes, Master."

"The energy on the opposite side of the circular flow is the heart and it is at its minimum when the liver is at its maximum. There are certain points on the body that influence the energy of each of the meridians. Martial artists have discovered these points because of the maximum amount of energy in the meridian and the minimum amount of energy in the meridian. When these points are touched, they have an immediate impact on the body." He paused.

"What time is it now?" he asked.

"About four in the afternoon," said Pei Ke. Liu nodded as he looked at the sun.

"At four in the afternoon, this point is tender and it will have an overall influence on the rest of the energy."

Liu touched the point and Pei Ke went immediately limp and fell to the ground. It was so fast, Pei Ke didn't even know what had happened.

"Master, what happened?"

"Do you know where I touched you?"

"Yes, Master."

The area was tender to the touch.

"Master, what is this point?"

"You need to remember what time of day it is and how I touched it. The point has some significance. It is not only the location of the point, but also how the point is touched. From what you already know you might be able to figure out some of the other points."

"Master, can you tell me where the other points are located?"

Liu smiled and walked off and Pei Ke followed, rubbing the spot where Liu had touched and wondering how to locate the rest of them. Liu had given him a clue: the secret to the point location had something to do with the time of day and where on the body the specific point was located. Maybe it was a certain classification of points. He knew there were connecting points and meeting points and other classifications of points.

As they walked, Pei Ke searched his mind to try to find the answer to his question. He fully understood why the information was not given out freely. It was one of those secrets a martial artist would keep to himself and only share with the most dedicated and loyal students. It is the custom of many martial artists to withhold some information from their students in case that the student ever challenged the teacher. Only those dedicated students who stayed with the teacher until he stopped teaching, would receive the most vital information at the very end of the teachers career. Liu was holding out a carrot, a hint of teaching to come, to make sure Pei Ke continued.

As he raced to catch up, he wondered if Liu had given the information to Wei Ken De. Wei Ken De had been with Liu for such a long time and Liu was soon going to stop teaching. He must have given him his final secrets. Pei Ke thought it might be appropriate for him to one day study with Wei Ken De, which of course made him think of Mei Li. He wondered what she was doing at that very moment.

He imagined Mei Li helping her father with his business, but he realized that he didn't know what business Wei Ken De was in. Maybe it was some sort of buying and selling. He certainly had free time to teach Mei Li, so it could not be too difficult. Maybe Wei Ken De would take him in as a student and he could learn the business. It would be a way to get closer to Mei Li.

Then he thought of Hua Yee. She was probably with Uncle Wu and taking care of the younger children. Not too exciting but it gave her the experience to be able to take care of a family. Mei Li, on the other hand, didn't have that experience.

As they walked, he compared the advantages of marrying each one of them. He concluded neither one was perfect and either one of them would forever enhance his future and fortune. He was lucky now; he didn't need to make a decision until sometime in the future.

# CHAPTER FIFTEEN

On the twelfth day, they woke and did their Qi Gong exercises as usual. When they had finished, Pei Ke turned to Liu and asked, "Master, why do women and men act differently?"

"Why do you ask me this? Doesn't your mind ever take a rest?"

Pei Ke looked at Liu, embarrassed. The question had come from nowhere, he knew.

"Are you planning on getting married in the near future?" Liu said.

"No, Master. I was just curious."

"Pei Ke, you have found there is a difference between the thought process of a woman and the thought process of a man. Is that correct?"

"Yes, Master. Why is that?"

"It is the question women ask about men. Are you asking which way of thinking is correct and which is incorrect?"

"I know you're going to say that neither is correct or incorrect, but I'd like to know why there is this difference."

"The answer is in the Universal Energy of the Tao. If you look at the symbol, you can see that each element of the symbol, the Yin and the Yang, both embraces and is embraced by the other. Individually, they are nothing, but together they are complete because they both embrace each other and keep each other in check.

"Women are, as you know, the Yin aspect and men are the Yang aspect and each has its own internal characteristics. There are things that make a woman a woman and there are things that make a man a man. These characteristics influence each other within the Yin and these characteristics influence each other within the Yang.

"For example, when a male has reached a certain age, he begins having secretions in his body that trigger a number of different factors, including his body, mind, and thought process. The same is true of a female. At a certain time in her life, there are secretions within her triggering certain female physical and mental characteristics.

"This is why there are differences between men and women. Neither is good or bad, as you rightly guessed. They are what they are and the difference should be celebrated, not seen as undesirable. Thus, you should celebrate the uniqueness of any woman you choose for a mate and she should do the same. If she can make you feel more like a man and you can make her feel more like a woman, then both of you have mastered a truly loving and strong relationship."

"Master, there have been many times that I've seen and heard of relationships that aren't like what you're describing. Why is that?"

"Pei Ke, you know that as an adult, I have not lived with a woman and I doubt I ever will. Thus, my conclusions are based solely on observation, but it seems the conflict between women and men comes from such things as a lack of respect and differences in each partner's expectations, wants and desires, and upbringing. Of course, there may be other elements, but to me, these seem to be predominant.

"This is why parents often select marriage partners for their children, rather than letting the children decide for themselves. Of course, there are often other motivations for that as well, such as economic security or to create political or military alliances. But for the common people, it is the experience of the family knowing how one would react within a social environment that leads to many of these decisions."

Pei Ke was uncertain where the conversation was going. He wanted to ask Liu some more questions but felt it might not be appropriate. He would save his questions for later.

# Chapter Sixteen

Pei Ke and Liu were walking around a slight bend in the road leading into a forested area when Pei Ke noticed movement to his right. As he turned his head towards it, he felt Liu grabbing his coat and pulling him to the opposite side of the road into a shallow depression. No sooner were they in the grassy area than they heard and saw arrows flashing overhead.

"Pei Ke we need to make it to the forest before they get too close. Follow me and run."

They both ran in the direction of the forest, staying in the depression, which gave them some measure of protection. As they ran, the arrows continued to come from the area across the road. Suddenly Liu stopped in his tracks as he looked into the forest. He saw those eyes looking at him, the same eyes he had seen before.

He caught his breath as he looked at the menacing sight. He could make out a human like shape, but it was the eyes that bothered him. He could see them even from such a great distance.

There was the usual sinister look about those eyes, and he wanted no part of it. As he stood there, he suddenly stumbled forward. Pei Ke almost bumped into him.

"Master we are almost to the forest. Why are we stopping? Master, let's go!"

Liu took a deep breath, looking once more at the dark shape and the eyes.

"No, Pei Ke," he said. "We need to make a stand here."

"What?" Pei Ke practically screamed. "Master, he has weapons and we don't. He can stay back twenty feet and just shoot us. Master, we need to go now!"

Fear grabbed Pei Ke in his chest. He felt he was going to urinate in his pants. Suddenly Liu grunted and grabbed his leg as an arrow grazed him. Blood started soaking through his pants.

"Master, you're hurt. Can you walk? I'll help you to the forest."

"No." Liu said firmly. He looked at Pei Ke. "Pei Ke, you must make a stand here. You must take care of this attacker. Give me the sack."

Pei Ke gasped as another arrow whizzed by.

"Master," he said frantically. "I don't know what to do. He has a bow and is shooting arrows at us. He is quickly coming toward us and will soon be on top of us. We don't stand a chance in this situation. I don't stand a chance."

Liu became stern and Pei Ke wondered wildly how he could be so calm with blood gushing down his leg.

"Pei Ke," he said. "Focus and don't panic. Breathe in slowly and calm your mind. Remember all that I have taught you."

Liu took a knife from his sleeve and gave it to Pei Ke.

"Take this," he said. "Now, get low so he can't see you and run twenty feet down this depression. When you're there, charge across the road towards the attacker yelling at the top of your voice. Keep running towards him for ten steps, than drop to the ground. As soon as you're on the ground, get up, and keep charging."

"Master?"

"No questions. Go now!"

Pei Ke did as he was told and ran down the depression. When he'd run twenty paces, he stood up and did exactly as Liu had told him. As he ran towards the attacker he held the knife in his right hand high above his head. He screamed at the top of his voice.

---

Bao looked at the two travelers. He knew who they were and what he had been paid to do. He had been waiting for hours for them to show up.

The cold had made him stiff in his fingers and feet. Now they were here and he was ready. He didn't feel the coldness now nor were his fingers stiff. He was ready to do what he had promised he could do.

Before staking out the location the night before, he made sure he had enough arrows in his quiver. He knew Liu's reputation and had no intention of trying to take him on at a close distance. He had nothing to lose.

He was close enough now that the next arrow would do more than just graze Liu's leg. Bao raised the bow and was about to release the arrow in Liu's direction when he heard the scream. He turned towards the scream and saw the boy running towards him. He turned towards Pei Ke, adjusted his bow, and took aim at Pei Ke.

Just as Bao released his grip on the arrow Pei Ke dived to the ground. The arrow was on target to Pei Ke, but the target had fallen down. Bao wasn't certain if he had hit the boy or the boy fell down before the arrow arrived. Bao grabbed another arrow from his quiver and adjusted the arrow. He turned towards Liu and took aim.

Another scream and momentarily he didn't know which target to shoot at. Liu and Pei Ke were closing from different directions. As Bao stepped sideways, he drew back the bow string to take aim at Liu. His foot slipped on the loose rocks and the arrow went wide of its target. He fell to the ground and was on one knee when Liu grabbed the bow and tossed it aside.

Bao jumped up and drew a knife from inside his shirt.

"Liu, you are going to die here and now," said Bao.

"I don't have a quarrel with you," said Liu. "Leave now. I know Chen Chang has sent you. Is it worth dying for something you will never get? He will never give you what he promised. Just leave us alone."

Bao looked at Pei Ke. The boy had a knife. Did he know how to use it? Bao looked at Liu and saw Liu was wounded from the arrow. His decision was to attack Liu. The wound would slow him down enough that he could kill Liu. Once Liu was dead, his job was finished.

Without further hesitation, he took the few steps forward to close the distance to Liu. He swung the knife back and forth in front of him to keep Liu at bay.

Pei Ke realized Liu was at a disadvantage. He leapt forward towards Bao and screamed at the top of his voice. As Bao turned, Liu took advantage of the distraction and closed the distance towards his opponent. With his hand, he grabbed Bao's hand to change the direction of the knife.

Bao turned into the force and tried to sweep his foot against Liu's wounded leg. Liu avoided the sweep and turned the knife towards Bao's chest. In the struggle, the two men went to the ground with Liu falling on top of Bao. Unintentionally, the knife went deep into Bao's chest penetrating his heart. Liu felt the body go limp and knew Bao had died instantly.

Liu stood up and looked into the surrounding forest. He saw the eyes that were always following him. Pei Ke looked in the direction Liu was looking.

"Master, is there someone else?"

"No, no one we need to worry about."

The eyes faded slowly and finally disappeared. Liu knew they would be back again but didn't know when. Liu looked down at Bao laying dead on the ground. It was truly a waste that he died.

"Master, we need to take care of your leg."

Liu looked down at his leg.

"It will be alright. The bleeding has stopped and I can walk. It doesn't hurt much. Let's go. Leave him here. Someone will find him and bury him."

Liu turned and walked away. Pei Ke noticed that Liu had a slight limp.

# CHAPTER SEVENTEEN

The fourteenth day, of their journey was no different than the previous days. The night before they had been lucky to find an accommodating farmer, who was willing to let them sleep in an extra room. The morning was cool but not so cold to prevent them from doing their Qi Gong exercises.

The farmer looked intently as Liu and Pei Ke were going through their routine. The farmer's wife came out a couple of times, but he quickly brushed her requests aside as he intently watched the master and student. When they had finished, the farmer hesitantly approached them. Liu motioned for him to approach.

"You are truly a master of Qi Gong," said the farmer. "I've seen others practicing it, but there is a quality of spirit or essence to what you do that I haven't seen before."

The farmer bowed to Liu and to Pei Ke.

"Have you ever had the opportunity to learn?" asked Liu.

"Many years ago, I was in Beijing and had the opportunity to visit with one of my friends. He had once lived in this area, but the life of farming was not suited to him, so he went to the big city to seek his fortune. After he had been there for a year, I received a letter from him inviting me to come and visit.

"Against my wife's wishes, I went to Beijing for a week. He was studying Qi Gong from a very famous Qi Gong master and introduced me to this teacher. I learned a few postures that way, but since I was not going to stay, and the master knew I was just visiting, he only briefly showed me the moves and did not elaborate on them.

"Watching you, I can easily see that I was taught movements, but not the essence of Qi Gong. Over the years, I have done the few movements I was taught, and I've gained a benefit from practicing them. I've often thought that there must be more to it than what I've learned. I see that some of the movements I know are very similar to the ones that you are doing. Would you be so kind as to critique the movements so that I can do them correctly?"

"Of course," Liu said. "Do the movements as you were taught and I will watch," said Liu.

Liu and Pei Ke watched as the farmer went through the movements. The farmer had not gone more than a few seconds before Pei Ke was overcome with gratitude that he was studying from Liu. He thought he could see every flaw in the farmer's movements. He wanted to jump up and make some corrections himself, but he knew Liu would be very upset if he did. When the farmer finished he looked at Liu.

"Good," said Liu. "The movements you've been taught are common among many systems of Qi Gong. You know the direction of the moves, but need just a little correction for you to gain more from your practice. In Qi Gong, just a small correction in the positioning of the body can mean a big change in the way the energy flows."

He turned to Pei Ke.

"Pei Ke I want you to help him correct his first movement."

Pei Ke was startled but pleased he was asked to help. He rose slowly and showed the farmer the movement he was doing. He noticed Liu watching in satisfaction and he grew more confident as he made the necessary corrections to the farmer's posture. Over the next ten minutes, Pei Ke made one adjustment after another to get the farmer's body in the proper position to tap into the Universal Energy.

"How do you feel now?" said Pei Ke.

"It's the same movement I've been doing all these years, but it is totally different than what I was doing. Before, I could feel a little energy, but now I can feel much more, especially in my hands and feet. In fact, it took me many minutes to feel the energy with the way I was doing Qi Gong, but now it comes readily and almost instantly. Young man, you have an exceptional teacher. He is giving you a gift you need to treasure for the rest of your life. It is a treasure no one can take from you and you can derive much joy and happiness from teaching others."

Pei Ke, somewhat embarrassed, turned to Liu. Liu nodded for him to continue. Pei Ke was showing the farmer the proper way to do the second posture when Liu came over.

"You have done well," said Liu to the farmer. "Unfortunately, we need to be on our way. We have a long distance to cover today and we want to get started before it gets too late. There is a chance that we will be coming back this way in the future. Would it be possible for one or both of us to stay with you on our return trip?"

"Of course," said the farmer. "It would be an honor for either one of you or both of you to stay with me for as long as you need. Thank you for correcting my form."

"How many more days till we get to Beijing?" asked Liu.

"If you make good time, it is another three days to Beijing. Let me give you my friends address. Maybe you can visit with him while you are there."

The farmer went inside and returned a minute or two later with a name and address scribbled on an old piece of rice paper. Liu looked at the writing and smiled to the farmer. The farmer had written the name of both his friend and his friend's teacher, along with both of their addresses. Liu recognized the name of the teacher. He had talked with him years previously when he had been in Beijing. Liu kept the information to himself but wondered if the man was still alive. It would be interesting to visit with him after all these years.

Liu and Pei Ke picked up their belongings and said good-bye to the farmer and headed out on the road towards Beijing. As they were walking, Pei Ke could see Liu was smiling.

"Master, thank you for letting me help that man."

"Did you learn anything from the experience?"

Pei Ke nodded.

"I tried to remember everything you've told me when I was showing him the correct way to do the postures."

"Do you feel more confident with the movements after having shown him how to do them correctly?"

"Yes, that is what I wanted to say. Somehow helping him actually helped me."

"You probably learned more than he did," said Liu.

They walked for about an hour and neither one of them said a word. Both were deep in thought. Finally Pei Ke turned to Liu.

"Master, can you elaborate on the concepts of Yin and Yang as they relate to disease. I know you have told me much about the subject, but I feel what I know is superficial compared to all that's out there."

"Pei Ke, the concept of Yin and Yang is very simple, as I have told you before. It is nothing more than complimentary opposites that have an influence on each other.

"While we walk, listen to what I say, but I also want you to do the following stepping pattern."

Pei Ke watched as Liu demonstrated the pattern he wanted Pei Ke to do.

"Master," said Pei Ke. "You've had me do this stepping pattern before."

"Foot techniques are vital for any type of martial arts. Each martial art has a unique pattern that should be mastered if you want to be good at the art. Hsing-Yi Chuan is no exception. Continue to do this stepping pattern. I will correct you as needed."

"Yes, Master."

"Now, think of Yin and Yang as the interplay between two opposing but complimentary forces. In Chinese medicine, there is the Yin aspect of a disease process and also the Yang aspect of a disease process. Knowing where the patient is in the disease process helps us to treat the disease. Treating a Yin disease process as if it was a Yang disease process will not help the patient at all, and in some instances can make the patient worse. Since most disease processes have both a Yin phase and a Yang phase, we need to be aware of both and determine which phase the patient is in at the time. Do you remember me telling you this before?"

"Yes, Master, I remember," said Pei Ke.

"You can think of the Yin and Yang aspect in many different ways. In martial arts, especially in Tai Chi Chuan there is the Yin aspect of the martial arts application and there is the Yang aspect of the martial art move. They flow from one to the other.

"Have you ever noticed that many times Tai Chi Chuan is represented by the Yin Yang symbol? The reason is the interplay in Tai Chi Chuan between the substantial and the insubstantial, fullness and emptiness, forward and backward, left and right, and up and down.

"I am going to give you an example now that not everyone agrees with. It is from my own experience and not the experience of others."

Pei Ke loved it when Master said such things. It made him feel special, like he was being initiated into some deep secret that only a few others had access to. He listened carefully.

For most of the rest of the day Liu showed Pei Ke how the movements of Tai Chi Chuan, and especially the martial arts applications, had both Yin and Yang aspects. When they finally started looking for a place to sleep, Pei Ke was exhausted.

# CHAPTER EIGHTEEN

The gods looked favorably on them that night. Once again, they found a place to stay without having to do extensive begging. A farmer and his wife were kind enough to take them in. After an early evening meal, the farmer was in a talkative mood.

"Master, it is fortuitous you have visited with us tonight. I was just telling my wife that I have had a pain in both wrists and arms for over two months now and it does not seem to go away. In fact, it is getting worse rather than better."

"What type of work do you do?" asked Liu.

"As you know I am a farmer, but I do very detailed leather stitching for the other farmers. The work is highly repetitive using my fingers, hands, and arms. My wrists are always in motion."

"Do you do this every day?"

"Not every day but often during the week. I am the only one who knows how to do this kind of work. The other farmers are relying on me to take care of their leather work."

"Do you have your hands close to your body when you do the work or are they always in front of you?"

"They are always in front of me."

"Show me where the pain is located."

Pei Ke watched as the man showed Liu the exact location of the pain on the wrist of his right hand and the radiating path up the inside of the forearm.

"If you give it some rest, does it feel better?" asked Liu.

"Yes, in the mornings it feels better, but by about mid-morning it starts to hurt again, and it hurts quite a bit by evening. If I hold my arm so as to immobilize the wrist, it seems to take some of the pressure and pain away, but I can't work that way all the time."

"Have you ever injured your arm, hand, or wrist?"

"No."

"Have you ever had the problem before?"

"No."

"Is it possible for you to discontinue doing that type of work?"

"This work and farming is all I know how to do, and I need to feed my family. If I don't work, we will have no money. My wife must stay home with the children. Everything is up to me."

Liu had the man sit so he could put his arm on the table and Liu could feel the pulses. Liu continued to ask many questions, following his typical diagnostic process. This included looking at the tongue and feeling the area where the man complained of the pain.

"Have you ever hurt your neck?" asked Liu.

"No."

"Have you ever been in any type of accident where there was a sudden jerking or snapping back and forth of your head or neck?"

"No."

"Have you ever injured your shoulder or elbow?"

"No."

"Please turn your neck to the left and then to the right."

The man did as he was instructed, and Liu noticed that the range of motion in turning to the left and right was different.

"Is it painful to turn your head left and right?"

"Yes, some. There is definitely more discomfort on one side versus the other. Why is that, do you think?"

"I think you have a blockage of energy in your neck, shoulder, or upper back, which is preventing the energy from flowing correctly from your neck to your wrist. This is what is causing you to have this pain."

"While I'm sitting here, there is no pain in my neck or shoulder, but there is pain in my wrist. Wouldn't the problem be in the area where the pain is located?"

"This is a common misconception many people and doctors have. It has led to many people being treated incorrectly. Frequently, the doctor will treat this problem and it will go away for a short time, only to come back. Quite often, a treatment such as this requires the patient to have his arm immobilized for an extended period of time, which, based on what you've said, is not an option for you."

"But how do you know for sure the problem is located in the neck?"

"You have pain in your wrist at this very moment, is that correct?"

"Yes."

"There are a couple of diagnostic procedures I do to help me determine if the problem is coming from the neck, shoulder, or upper back. May I press on some acupuncture points to help me isolate the problem?"

"Of course."

Liu held the top of man's head with his left hand and put his fingers of his right hand on the man's neck. Liu gently turned the man's neck as he applied pressure to selected areas of the neck. Liu could feel certain muscles of the neck that had gone into spasm, causing the muscle to become knotted. Liu searched for the exact location that would give him his answer and gently pressed on the point.

"Master, where you are pressing is very sore."

Liu then shifted to the left side and did the same thing on the left side of the man's neck. He could find no corresponding knotted muscle. The knotted muscle only existed on the right side. Liu went back to this special point on the right side.

"I am going to push a little harder on this. Try not to jerk or turn your head. I will be applying more pressure."

Liu pressed on the point and held it for a moment. He gently released his grip of the neck and head.

"How does your wrist feel now?"

The man moved his hand and wrist, turning it in different directions.

"How did you do that? The pain in my wrist and forearm is much better."

"Do you now think the problem exists in your wrist or in your neck?"

"Based on what you just did, it is obvious the problem is in my neck. Is it just that simple? I press on the point and the problem will go away?"

"No, it is highly unlikely that simply pressing the point will cause the pain to go away completely. What I would like to do is press on some more points to help me determine how to treat this problem. I want you to stand up and put your hands on my upper back."

The man did as Liu had asked. Liu guided him to the exact location on his upper back that he wanted the man to put his hands.

"Now, I want you to watch what I do with my arms."

Liu put his right hand on his left shoulder and his left hand on his right shoulder.

"What do you notice happening with my shoulder blades now that my hands are on the opposite shoulder?"

The man thought for a while and then said, "Can we do it again?"

Liu dropped his hands and again placed his hands on the opposite shoulders.

"The shoulder blade moves away from the spine," said the man.

"Correct. Now there is a wider space between the spine and the shoulder blade. I want you to sit in the chair."

After the man got seated, Liu pressed on the man's upper back."

"Painful?" asked Liu.

"It is a little uncomfortable, but not really painful."

"I want you to put your hands on your opposite shoulders like you saw me do."

The man did as he was instructed. Liu pressed on the upper back and the man winced in pain.

"I assume where I am pressing is painful."

"Yes, it is very painful. Why is the point so painful?"

"It is painful because the energy in your body is blocked someplace, causing the muscles in this area to go into spasm. It is the same with the sore points on your neck."

"If you press on those points like you did with my neck will it help with the pain in my wrist and forearm?"

"Maybe," said Lu. "It depends on where and how the energy is blocked. From my experience pressing on either point can help or pressing on both points can help. In some instances, pressing on one point can make it worse and the other makes it better. We just have to try. Regardless of which one works and which one does not work, it is my opinion that the pain in your wrist and forearm is not due to a problem with the nerves in your wrist; rather, it is a problem with the blockage of energy in your neck and upper back. Treating the wrist will only give you temporary relief and, sooner or later, the neck and upper back will need to be treated."

"Can you fix the problem for me?" asked the man.

"I would need to do acupuncture and you will need to have a series of treatments. I can do the first treatment, but you would need to find someone else to continue with the other treatments. In addition, I want you to find someone to press on the points on your upper back every day. Do not do the neck points. There is a special technique for doing this and if it is done wrong the patient can be hurt. Do you understand?"

"Yes," said the man. "My son can press on the points for me."

"Pei Ke, do you understand how I diagnosed this problem?"

"Yes, Master."

Liu motioned for the man to lie on the bed. He positioned the man's legs and arms in a special way to allow the needles to be inserted at the correct depth and angle. In this treatment, the angle was crucial, both for the safety of the patient and for maximum efficiency.

The first two needles Liu inserted were in Shen Mai and Hou Xi acupuncture points. Liu explained that the combination of points were part of the Turtle Point combinations and when used together had a positive effect on the upper back, neck, and shoulders. Shen Mai was, he explained particularly effective in treating neck stiffness due to wind problems. Hou Xi, on the other hand, was particularly effective in treating scapular pain. Together, they treated the area from the neck to the scapular. It was a very effective combination.

"Pei Ke, do you have any questions on how this patient was treated?"

"Not so much with the treatment, Master. But what if his problem with his wrist turned out not to be his neck? How would you have treated him?"

"I would have tried to determine which meridian in the area of his wrist was either in excess or deficiency, and then I would try to balance the energy in the affected meridian.

"Of course, that is a simple answer," said Liu. "The balancing process can be difficult though. The problem could be associated with a particular meridian or there could be an imbalance in the meridian running through the wrist. Is this too confusing for you?"

"No, I understand. The problem the doctor faces is trying to determine which meridian or meridians are causing the problem. It is very likely that the meridian closest to the problem is causing the pain, but it could also be another meridian."

"Yes, and that is where Five Element and the Mother-Son theories we've talked about before are very important in the diagnostic process. The Mother-Son Theory can become very confusing unless you have studied it for some time. It becomes more confusing when it is expanded further to encompass more relationships between meridians."

"Can you explain this to me further?" said Pei Ke.

"I will," Liu said. "But now it is too early in your learning process. I will share this information with you at a later time, when it will mean more to you."

"Yes, Master. I understand."

"Now the technique you just saw can also be used to treat elbow pain. Elbow pain is sometimes a repetitive motion problem existing in the scapular area and the neck, rather than in the elbow, just as we have seen here. It comes about quite often when people need to swing items like a scythe or other farming implements. Sometimes the implement will hit the ground, and the vibrations of the impact go up the implement into the arm and affect the scapular and neck. Again, it is possible to solve these problems by using the technique I have just used. Do you have any questions about treating these types of problems?"

While Pei Ke was thinking about what to ask next, Liu turned to the farmer.

"Are you alright?" asked Liu. "You seem to be watching very intently."

"It is all so fascinating," said the farmer. "We need someone like you to stay and help take care of us farmers."

"There is always a need for more doctors. Maybe someone in this area could go to Beijing and study and then come back to take care of everyone."

As the farmer was pondering what to say next, Liu turned to Pei Ke.

"Master, from what you told me while we were traveling to your ancestral home, it would be possible to treat a wrist and elbow pain problem by finding the corresponding sore point on the opposite leg."

"Yes, it would be possible, but from my experience, using the corresponding point on the leg would be more effective if it were actually a problem with the wrist. In our patient here, it is a neck problem causing the wrist pain and not a problem with the wrist."

"Master, if his problem was a wrist problem due to an injury to the wrist, would it be advisable to put a needle directly into the area where there is pain?"

"In general, you are correct," said Liu. "Experience and some common sense factors will guide you in this decision. In this case, if it were a wrist problem I would have asked him to point to the location on the wrist where the pain was the greatest. It would be at this point, along with others based on the differential diagnosis, that I would put a needle.

"I might also apply some moxibustion to the needle to enhance the effect of the treatment. Of course, if there were some indication of heat or swelling in the area then I wouldn't apply the heat."

"Why wouldn't you apply heat if there were indication of heat or swelling?"

"While there are always exceptions, my philosophy is that I don't apply heat to a problem that already has heat. This concept can be used for both external problems like joints and also for internal problems especially when you are putting together an herbal formula. It also is applicable for boils and abscesses.

"It would also be something you would want to consider any time there is an excess condition, since the moxibustion has a tendency to tonify, or increase, the energy. In terms of excess conditions, you generally want to disperse energy rather than increase energy. In some instances, when you increase energy to an excess condition you make the problem worse.  Do you understand?"

"Yes, Master."

Pei Ke thought for a moment before asking. "I know I will be off our current topic, but can I ask a question?"

"Yes, ask the question," interrupted the farmer. I don't understand everything you have said but it is interesting."

"Master, I know I have asked this question at least twice before. In general, how do you identify excess and deficiency conditions?"

"The question needs to be asked in context of the differentiation of syndromes as it applies to exterior and interior, cold and hot, and Yin and Yang. But to give you a basic answer, heat, redness, brightness, yellowness, and swelling are excess conditions. Cold, white, paleness, and contraction are deficiency conditions. These are only a few of the ways to distinguish between excess and deficiency, and they relate to what you can see visibly. In Traditional Chinese Medicine, an imbalance of energy can be summed up as either an excess or deficiency or both. Solve the imbalance and you have started a healing process for the patient.

"In general, we as doctors can heal nothing. All we do is balance the energy in the body so the body can utilize its own capacity to heal itself. Our responsibility to our patients and ourselves is to make the patient whole based on our education, knowledge, experience, and abilities. Above all, do the patient no harm. This is a big responsibility for both of us. Do you have more questions?"

"Yes, Master," said Pei Ke. "Are there more of these Turtle point combinations you just demonstrated?"

"Yes, there are actually four pairs or combinations affecting different areas of the body. Since you have asked, I will explain them to you in detail.

"I have already explained the combination of Shen Mai and Hou Xi. The combination of Nei Guan on the arm and Gong Sun on the foot is useful in treating problems and diseases of the heart, chest, upper abdomen, and stomach. In my clinical experience, this combination is useful anytime a patient complains of problems of the upper abdomen or chest. It doesn't have to be a disease process. It can be an injury or any chest congestion.

"The combination of Wai Guan on the inside of the forearm and Zu Lin Qi on the outside of the foot is effective for those problems on the cheek and the outer edge of the eye. From my clinical experience, this combination is also good for treating digestive problems.

"The combination of Lieh Que on the arm by the wrist and Zhao Hai located below the inside part of the ankle bone is effective for treating problems of the throat, chest, and lungs.

"These four combinations also have a very soothing effect on the body. Many times patients will indicate their whole body relaxes when these combinations are used. I have found in clinical experience that using Qi Gong in combination with acupuncture on these points substantially enhances the effect of the treatment. Of course, you can use other points when you use these combinations."

"Master, when you use these Turtle points do you tonify or disperse the energy?"

"Since these points are used in combination, you will want to decide what condition the patient has and then, based on the pulses, determine if the treatment process would be better suited to tonification or dispersion. I know this does not answer the question, but it is a question I cannot give a general answer to."

Pei Ke thought for a moment and was about to ask another question when Liu looked at him.

"Don't be confused. There is a reason I am giving this information to you in small portions. It would not be possible for anyone to absorb everything at once. Remember, it took thousands of years and generations of doctors to piece this information together. You can't learn it all at once."

Pei Ke nodded. He realized that each generation contributed more information to this large body of knowledge. Pei Ke wondered what Liu had contributed. He was sure some of it was in the small scrolls Liu always carried in the sack. It must be as he indicated before, priceless information people would be willing to kill for.

"Pei Ke, enough questions, we need to treat this patient."

# CHAPTER NINETEEN

Pei Ke realized the more he learned the more he wanted to learn, but even though he liked the concept of studying from Liu, it was daunting to think that he was making a life-long commitment. He wondered how any one person could have learned so much as his teacher. When did Liu ever have time to do anything else but study? Maybe he studied just for the sake of studying. Pei Ke wondered if Liu had ever had any feelings for a woman. He wondered how he was going to ever ask him the question.

"Master you've been studying for most of your life. Do you ever get bored?"

Liu smiled.

"No, I find it very gratifying to continually study. Even though I do not now have teachers, I enjoy reviewing and improving on what I already know. I really wish my teachers were still alive. There are so many questions I could ask them now that I am proficient in these arts.

"It is always a challenge for me to improve. This is true for not only the martial arts but also for the calligraphy, painting, and poetry. It is such a pleasure for me to totally immerse myself in each one of these arts. Hopefully, you will also see the advantages of my life long study and some day impart to others what I am imparting to you. It takes time to learn, but you must continually practice and practice hard to become proficient."

Pei Ke thought about what Liu had just said. It would indeed be many years of study and practice, but the rewards would be great and it would never be boring. There would always be a challenge with each new patient. He was indeed very lucky that Liu was so willing to share his knowledge.

"Master, you have taught me basically how to take the pulses and I have been feeling my pulses routinely. When you have allowed me to take the pulse of a patient I have paid attention to the twenty eight different pulses. Can you give me some more information about the pulses?"

"As I have mentioned to you before, the taking of the pulses is one of the most difficult techniques to master, and it takes a lifetime of continual practice to really be good at it. Some of the true masters of pulse taking can tell you many things about what has taken place in your body over the years. Knowing what has happened to a person previously will help the doctor determine how to treat existing health care situations.

"If you remember, I told you a normal pulse is smooth in nature, even in its consistency, and has about four heart beats per breath. Of course, you have to take into consideration a number of factors when you take the pulse. You would expect the pulses to be slower with an athlete, weaker with an elderly person, faster with a woman who is pregnant, and exaggerated with someone who is under a lot of emotional strain. As an example, if there were two men alongside of each other and one was an athlete and the other was elderly and they only had the difference of a slow pulse you might make a wrong decision based solely on the pulses. The age of each person needs to be taken into consideration."

"What should I look for first when taking the pulses?"

"Everyone who teaches pulse diagnosis has a different opinion. In my opinion, the first thing you should do is to distinguish between fast and slow. This is probably the easiest one to distinguish. Once this is done, then you should distinguish between a deep and superficial pulse. In other words, does the pulse feel like it is close to your fingers or is it farther away. The third thing is to distinguish between the pulses being excess or deficient.

"This will cover six of the twenty-eight different pulses and is the first step in trying to understand the pulses. If you can do this, then you are ready to tackle the next characteristics of the pulse taking."

"Is it possible for me to take the pulses of more of your patients after you have taken their pulses?"

"If it is appropriate, I will let you do it."

"Master, it seems what you just told me is basically the differentiation of Yin and Yang."

"Yes, you can think of it that way."

"Master, it seems to me that this is true with other diagnostic methods as well, such as the Eight Principles."

"Yes. Many of the signs and symptoms you see are common sense when you understand Yin and Yang. If you had a patient with a slow pulse, would you expect it to be Yin or Yang?"

"As you've told me before, Yin is cold, withdrawn, slow, depleted, deficiency, and interior. So, if a patient had a slow pulse, I would expect a Yin factor of some kind. Of course, based on our previous conversations, I would need to know a little more about the person and I expect that would come from a detailed intake of the patient's history and other factors in the diagnostic process."

"Good."

Pei Ke thought about what he had just said. He was formulating a question when Liu spoke.

"If all you knew about a patient is they were Yin in nature, would you want to make the person more Yin or Yang?"

"If the person was Yin and that means something is cold, depleted, and deficient along with some other characteristics then I would want to change the Yin to make the person less Yin."

"Think of Yin and Yang as each being a cup of liquid. When each cup is half full, it has the appropriate amount. Yes, they are opposites, but a person can also have a deficient amount of Yin in one meridian and an excess amount of Yang in another meridian at the same time. It would be better to change the deficient amount of Yin and bring it back to its normal state. Increasing the Yang may do as much harm as depleting a deficient Yin. That is enough information for now. Think about it for a while and then ask me at a later time if you still don't understand."

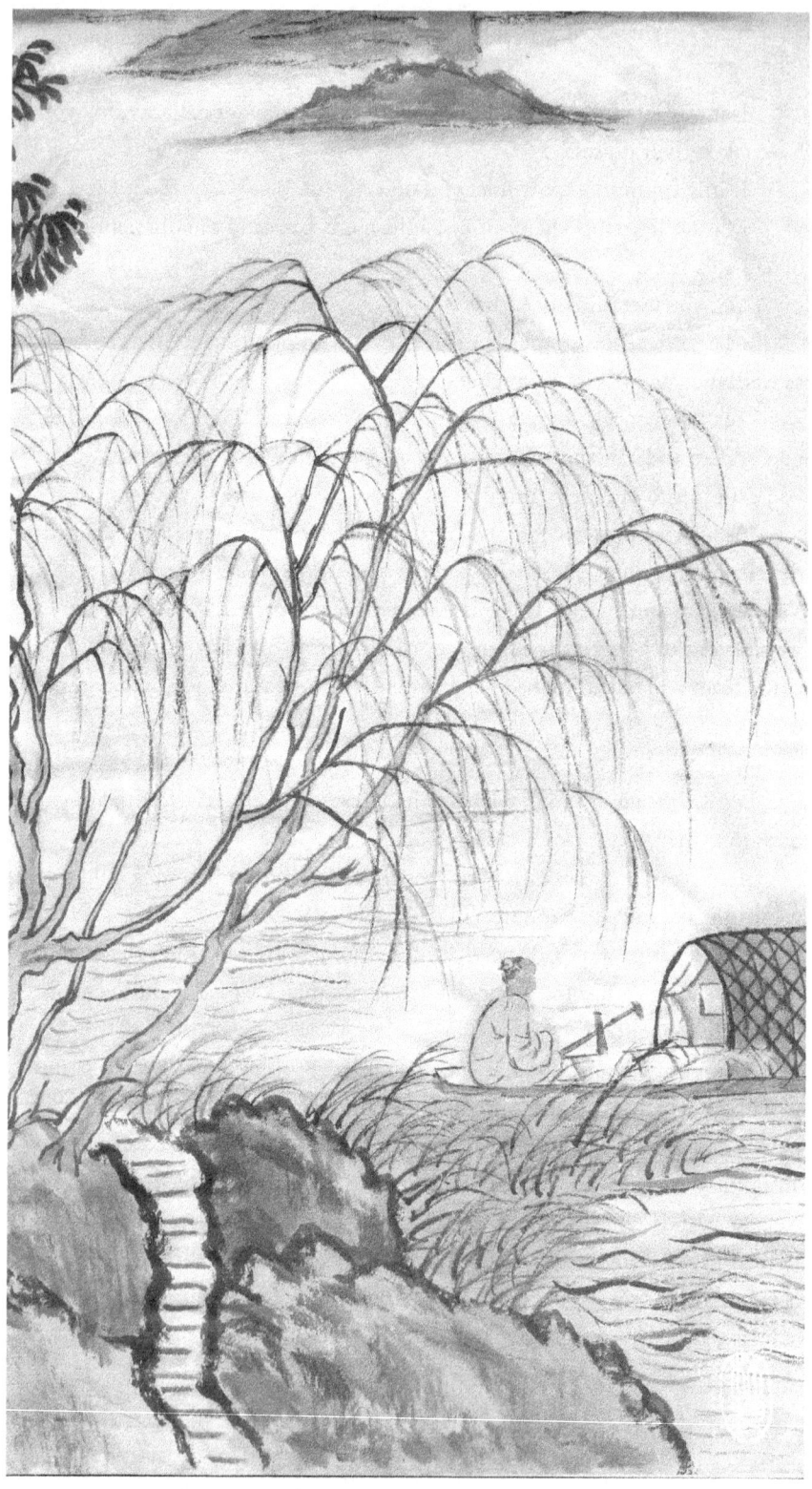

# CHAPTER TWENTY

The early morning sun shone brightly as they continued on their journey. The night before they had found a small temple located near a secluded lake. The resident monks had welcomed them as was the custom and provided for their food and shelter needs.

"Master."

"Yes."

"Quite some time ago you told me for each one of our organs in our body, there is a meridian associated with it. Is one organ and its associated meridian more important than another?"

"The Zang-Fu organs are composed of both the Yin and Yang organs of our body, and thus we have Yin and Yang meridians. Each one of the organs and meridians has a specific function within the body. Not only does the organ affect the meridian but, as I explained to you before, the meridian affects the organ. If we were missing one of the organs, then a specific function within our body is compromised and the energy of the organ is somewhat compromised.

"How it effects an individual will vary based on first the health of the other organs, then the functioning of the other meridians, and finally the constitution of the person. This is readily seen when you look at the Five Element Theory where there are the constructive and destructive cycles of the flow of energy.

"It would be incorrect for me to say one organ and meridian is better or more important than another. It is the overall working of the total system, with all meridians in harmony with each other that gives us our optimum health. However, we can say there are certain organs that the body can function without and others that it cannot.

"It is possible to live without a gallbladder. Your quality of your life would not be at its optimum, but you could survive. However, it is not possible to function without a heart.

"In Traditional Chinese Medicine, the heart has three basic characteristics. First, it is the organ propelling the blood through our body. If the Qi of the heart is strong and vigorous, the pulse you feel on the radial artery on the Cun position of the left hand will be regular and vibrant.

"Now, Pei Ke, if the heart Qi is deficient what would you expect to find on the pulse?"

Pei Ke thought for a moment.

"I would expect the heart Qi to be weak."

"Yes, you are correct. It would also feel a little thready."

"Master, what is a thready pulse? You have mentioned this a couple of times in the past. I should have asked you before."

"A thready pulse is clear and distinct, but feels like a fine piece of thread. It is an indication of a deficiency in the body due to Qi and Blood deficiency. We see this in patients who might have had a prolonged illness.

"In addition to the pulse, the patient's complexion would be different based on the strength of the Qi in the heart. If the heart Qi is strong, then the person will have a lively complexion. Sometimes it might even look like it glows. If the heart Qi is weak or deficient, then the face will look pale or bland, and it will lack a sense of being alive."

"Master, that means anytime I see someone I can enhance my diagnosis by looking at the persons face."

"Yes, face reading is an art, but you have to be careful. You will need to know more about the other organs and how they affect the face for you to make an accurate diagnosis. As an example, when someone has a yellow tint to their face, this might be an indication of a liver organ problem and not a heart problem."

Pei Ke thought about this. Once again, it was the combination of signs and symptoms that lead to the correct diagnosis, not just once a single sign or symptom.

"The second characteristic you need to be familiar with concerning the heart is the mind. Our mental activities and our overall mental balance are associated with the well being of the heart Qi. Since the heart is associated with the flow of blood and the blood goes to our head and mind, then there is a correlation between the two. One way to think about it is to think of the heart as the seat or center of our emotions."

"Master, occasionally there are times when my mind doesn't seem right. Is this what you're talking about?"

"I would need to know more specifics but, in general, you are correct. However, if someone told me they were depressed and angry all the time, I would consider a liver energy imbalance. It is possible, however, that both a heart and a liver energy problem exist.

"The third characteristic would be that the heart Qi opens to the tongue. In other words, in Traditional Chinese Medicine there is a energetic connection between the heart and the tongue. If a patient told me they couldn't taste the food they eat, then I might suspect it is an imbalance in the heart Qi.

"Knowing what you now know about Yin and Yang, what color would you suspect the tongue to be if there was an excess condition in the Qi?"

"The tongue would be brighter. With a deficiency condition, the tongue would be pale in color."

"Good. Remember when I told you about the tongue and the parts of the body that are associated with areas of the tongue? I told you the tip of the tongue is associated with the heart. If there was an excess condition then I would expect the tip of the tongue to be redder than the rest of the body of the tongue. In addition, deep cracks along the center line of the tongue leading to the tip may be indicative of a heart organ and or heart Qi problem."

"Master, this is a lot of information. Am I right in assuming that each of our organs has the same wealth of information to remember?"

"Yes, you are correct. If I tell you all there is to know about the heart right now you will not remember it. What I have given you is just a small amount of what you need to know. I don't want you to feel overwhelmed. It takes a lot of study to remember this information about the heart, and as you say, each one of our organs has specific information similar to what you have just learned about the heart. For now, I just want you to remember the heart. Later we will take each of the other organs and analyze them.

"But there is one more piece of information I want you to remember. There are relationships between the organs. Remember a few minutes ago I mentioned the relationship between the liver and the heart? Well, there are similar relations between the heart and lung, heart and spleen, heart and kidney, spleen and lung, liver and lung, lung and kidney, liver and spleen, spleen and kidney, and liver and kidney."

"Does each of those relationships have its own unique qualities?

"Yes, but it is better to say indications than to say qualities. Let's take the heart-liver relationship. The heart can be referred to as the 'seat of our emotions.' Remember, at the start of this journey, we went to visit Mrs. Wang? Her problem was Liver Fire Rising. Do you remember her symptoms?"

"She had headaches and felt lethargic and depressed."

"The liver energy problem had affected her emotions. In Traditional Chinese Medicine, the heart is in control of blood and the liver stores the blood. If there is a deficiency of heart energy, then the liver cannot store it properly and satisfy the needs of the physical body. When there is an imbalance of the heart energy, it can lead to an imbalance of the liver energy, giving rise to the patient experiencing palpitations, insomnia, and eye problems. When there is excess of liver Qi, it affects the heart giving rise to problems such as headache and mental restlessness."

"I am going to guess each one of these relationships has its own specific health care issues when there is an imbalance."

"Yes," said Liu. "You are correct. In addition, there is a relationship between the coupled meridians and organs. The order of the flow of energy follows the coupling of the meridians. For every Yin meridian there is a Yang meridian. The order of the flow of energy is lung, large intestine, stomach, spleen, and so on. Do you remember?"

"Yes."

"The lung and large intestine relationship is a good example. Lung is Yin in nature and large intestine is Yang and they follow each other in the energy cycle.

"When the lung energy does not work correctly, then there may be an effect on the large intestine energy. When the large intestine energy does not work correctly, then there may be an effect on the lung energy."

"As you can see, we are an interrelated system where an imbalance in one place in the body can affect another place. The effect is entirely dependent on the constitution of the individual. As an example, let's suppose three individuals each have a blockage of energy on the Lung Meridian and in each case it can be classified as an excess. Let's also say the blockage is of the same intensity for all three and the pulse of the Lung Meridian is the same for all three. With just that information, the patient can manifest three different symptoms, and the problem can be manifested not only on the Lung Meridian but also on another meridian.

"Women seem to be more aware of how this can happen than men. Ask any woman if, when something goes wrong with one part of her body, it affects another part of her body. Almost every woman will say yes. To them it is like a cascade effect. One thing goes wrong and then another thing goes wrong. Of course, those who are associated with her may think she is making up these complaints, but to her they are real. And it is true; these complaints are real.

"It is a circular effect for the patient. One thing leads to another, which leads to another. After a while the patient is awash in complaints and becomes overwhelmed by the whole process. Each day can be different. One day one complaint is worse, and she is focused on that complaint for a while until another one of the complaints seems the most important. It is a circular series of complaints. It is our responsibility to find out where the root of the problem exists in this circular series of energy blockages and complaints.

"The doctor who treats each complaint separately or who refers the patient to a series of 'specialists' to address each complaint, can easily put the patient on a never ending round of doctors. You must be able to use your skills to find the root cause of the energy imbalance and solve it.

"A good intake exam is crucial when you first meet the patient. It is easy for you to overlook one of the complaints because the patient either was focused on one problem or forgot to mention some of the other problems. Remember, when we treated Mrs. Wang? If she only gave me some of the information and I did not pry the other information from her, then I might have diagnosed the problem wrong, and of course, the treatment protocol would not have been as effective."

"In other words, you are telling me some patients withhold information."

"Yes, they may withhold information because they feel embarrassed about it, or they may have simply forgotten it, or they don't think it's relevant. Remember, the patient is usually focused on the most severe problem at the moment.

"It is best for you to tell the patient you can only make a good diagnosis if you have all the information. Make sure they understand they are to tell you everything, even what they may consider the most unimportant piece of information, and you are the one to sort through the information to find what is relevant and what is not relevant.

"It might help to give them an example of Liver Fire Rising and Liver Blood Deficiency. Only a few symptoms separate the diagnosis of the two conditions. If one piece of information is missing, then the diagnosis is wrong and the treatment may not be effective."

"How do you know the patient has told you all the information about his or her condition?"

"This comes from experience. There are many different correlations in Traditional Chinese Medicine. If the patient tells me one thing, then I would expect the patient would tell me something else. As an example, if the patient were to tell me their knee hurt, I need to know how they hurt their knee. It could be because of a true knee injury or it could be an indication there is a lower back issue and the problem is actually in the back and not in the knee.

"Treating the knee for the pain may help a little, but if the problem is a blockage of energy in the lower back affecting the gall bladder, bladder, or kidney, then I should concentrate on the back. This is where it would be appropriate to ask the patient if there is pain in the lower back or if they have ever had a lower back injury. If you can rule out the back then you can concentrate on another cause for the knee problem."

Liu went on to explain more correlations. As he explained more, Pei Ke could feel his brain being filled to its capacity.

# CHAPTER TWENTY-ONE

"Master," asked Pei Ke. "If someone attacks me by grabbing my arm or clothes, what do I do?"

Liu thought for a moment before answering the question. He had been asked the question by other students and, based on the level of development of the student he had a different answer for each student. Usually, he asked the student to show him a grab and Liu would be able to release the grab, but that did not help the student learn, since there are an unlimited number of grabs one might need to defend against. Pei Ke's development was progressing to the point where he felt Pei Ke could understand the answer.

"Pei Ke, you asked me the same question before and I showed you some techniques."

"Yes, Master. I know, but can you give me more information and show me some more advanced techniques?"

"Your response to the grab depends on whether or not the person intends to do you harm. I assume you are referring to a situation where someone is intending to hurt you. Is that correct?"

"Yes, Master."

"Pei Ke, grab my right wrist."

"What kind of grab do you want me to use?"

"It doesn't matter. Just grab me."

Pei Ke grabbed Liu's right wrist with his left hand.

"I want you to grab me as if you were attacking me. Your grab is very weak."

Pei Ke grabbed again and held on as tight as he could. As soon as his fingers were closed tightly around Liu's wrist, Pei Ke felt pain shooting up his arm. Liu's movement to escape the grab was so fast Pei Ke didn't even see what happened.

"There are literally hundreds of Chin Na techniques and methods," Liu said. "Learning those techniques are good, but you need to know more than just some techniques. Many of these techniques are only useful if the situation is just right for their use. If one or more variables change, such as a slight shift of an arm position or a slight variation in the grab, then quite often you cannot execute the intended move.

"I want you to review and practice some of the basic Chin Na principles so that you will be able to extricate yourself from unwanted situations. Do you remember what I taught you before about joints?"

"Yes, Master. I remember."

"Good. Then you will recall that force is usually linear in direction and intensity. Linear force can quite often be defeated with circular movements. Hold on to my wrist with the same intensity you did before."

Pei Ke did as he was told, anxiously waiting for the intense pain to go up his arm. He watched as Liu redirected the force with a circular movement of his arm.

"Pei Ke, now I am going to grab your arm."

As soon as Liu had grabbed Pei Ke's arm, Liu could feel Pei Ke's arm and body become tense and started to struggle to get out of the grab. Liu released the grab.

Pei Ke was amazed at how strong Liu was. The grab actually hurt, and he felt his arm become immobilized right on the spot. There was no way he could get out of the grab no matter how strong he was.

"Pei Ke, grab my arm again, just like I grabbed yours."

Pei Ke grabbed and held on as hard as he could. With little or no effort, Liu was out of the grab.

"Master, what if I held on with the other hand?"

"You can try," said Liu.

The same thing happened. Liu used little or no effort to escape.

"Master, what if I held on at a different spot on your arm?"

Liu extended his arm and Pei Ke instantly grabbed and pulled as hard as he could. In a fraction of a second, Pei Ke was lying flat on the ground with his arm in an arm lock and Liu applying pressure to it.

Liu grabbed Pei Ke and yanked him to his feet.

"Are you all right?" asked Liu.

"Master, you could have easily broken or dislocated my shoulder!"

"Yes, I could have, if I had wanted to. Another ounce or two of pressure and I would have a student with a dislocated shoulder or broken collar bone."

Pei Ke rubbed his sore shoulder as the two of them stared at each other. Anger raced through Pei Ke's mind as he tried to get the pain out of his shoulder.

"The learning process is not always pleasant," said Liu. "I often inwardly cursed my teachers. I stayed with them because even though they seemed mean at times, they had my best interest at heart. Today I miss them a lot and wish I could meet with them to ask a million questions."

"Master, I still want to know how you did that."

"You need to know the following. This is in addition to what I already told you about Chin Na. The body has to be rooted to the ground. This will help you to turn on your center line and redirect the force. The force coming to you is linear in nature so the best way to defeat linear force is with circular motion. When the force is applied, you need to be aware of the position of your opponent's hand. You should be centered to the force and, whenever possible, turn into the force. If you can't turn into the force because of your position, then you need to turn away from the force. The primary consideration, though, is to turn into the force.

"You must know where the opponent has both hands. You can usually feel both hands or by the position of his body know where the hands are located. Quite often when someone grabs you with one hand, the other hand is free to hit you. You want to make sure you can block or disable the opponent before they can attack further.

"One of the best ways to get out of a Chin Na move or grab is to remember the principles of Pa Kua Chang. The coiling action and especially the twisting and turning of the arms and legs will put you into a favorable position."

As they walked along the road Liu continued explaining principles and concepts needed to effectively neutralize almost any type of force.

"Now that you know some more about Chin Na and force neutralization, I want you to start practicing on yourself. I know it is not the same as if you had a partner, but it will help you to ingrain it in your mind. Watch what I do."

Pei Ke watched as Liu took one hand and grabbed the other hand. Liu would counter the grab by turning and twisting to neutralize his own grab. It looked like someone was manipulating a puppet on the stage. It looked funny at first, but Liu slowed down the movements and Pei Ke could see where pressure was being applied against acupuncture points, joints and muscles.

Then, without warning Liu turned quickly and grabbed Pei Ke's hand with as much force as he could. Pei Ke felt the intensity of the grab and immediately tightened the muscles in his body and started to pull away. No matter how hard he pulled, he could not get away. Finally, Liu let him go.

"What did you do wrong?"

"Master, your grab was painful."

"And I suppose that when others grab you it will not be painful? Now what did you do wrong?"

"You caught me by surprise."

"Ah. So your enemies will announce their intentions so that you will have time to prepare? Now Pei Ke, stop making excuses. Think about what you just did when I grabbed you. Let me know when you have an answer."

Liu and Pei Ke continued along the road towards Beijing with Pei Ke deep in thought. The pain in his arm was still there, but he did as Liu had told him. He grabbed one wrist with the other hand and noticed the directions the wrist would turn and what directions caused him discomfort. He realized this process was a process of discovery.

# CHAPTER TWENTY-TWO

On the nineteenth day Liu and Pei Ke had taken breakfast with a family who had befriended them the day before. They had been traveling and had needed a place to stay for the night. Liu had walked past numerous buildings. From the outside, it was easy to tell that some of the houses he saw were occupied by people who had a considerable amount of wealth.

There were also many houses where the inhabitants were obviously not so well off. Liu approached one of the houses where it was obvious the occupants lacked the finer things in life. He asked if there was a place for them to sleep for the night. The farmer was a little hesitant until Liu had explained that they were willing to sleep anywhere and were willing to do some work in exchange for food and a sleeping area.

"Master," Pei Ke said the next morning, when they'd continued their journey. "I didn't want to ask last night while we were staying with the farmer and his wife, but of all the places you could have asked to stay, you chose the place which seemed to be the least desirable. Why was that?"

"Did you have enough to eat last night?"

"Yes, Master, there was plenty to eat. It wasn't elaborate food but it was enough. In fact, it tasted very good."

"We helped the farmer while we were there. You chopped wood, and I helped his wife with some of her health care issues. We gave value for value.

The farmer felt good about helping us and we felt good about helping them. We both felt relaxed. Would you have felt as good as you now feel if you had stayed at a place that was very opulent?"

Pei Ke thought for a few moments before answering. It was true; he felt at ease with the family they stayed with. The farmer and his family were simple but very genuine. There was nothing artificial with their behavior, and the couple, along with their children seemed to be very happy.

"Master, I was comfortable staying there even though the accommodations they gave us were very meager. The food, as you indicated, was enough and it tasted good. The farmer seemed to be happy we stayed with them and even told us we were welcome again if we ever returned to the area. If we were to stay somewhere more comfortable, more lavish, maybe the hospitality would not be the same. Why is that?"

"People are more comfortable with others if there is a commonality between them. We appear not to have anything and the farmer did not feel he was allowing a different class of people into his home. What he did not realize is we have more than he has but in riches he cannot comprehend. In his mind, he has the greater riches, even though he is poor. In his mind, he is above us but not by much and that made him comfortable.

"If we were to stay with a wealthy family they might not want us to stay in their house. They would have us stay with the servants. The servants would give us food, but would not interact with us. Granted, it would appear to us we were staying in a luxurious place, but in reality it would not be luxurious for us."

"What if we went to a well-to-do family and you told them who you were. Certainly, it would make a difference."

"It would make a difference only if they had heard about my family, which is unlikely. Why would they believe me without an introduction from someone else?

"The farmer and his family were happy even though they did not have money. So it is not the money that makes one happy. It is not the accumulation of physical items that makes one happy. It is the interaction one has with the Tao or Universal Energy that makes one happy. Now you know why I chose to stay where we stayed."

"Master, your family must have been happy, and they had a considerable amount of wealth."

"Yes, but it was not always the case. The wealth accumulated by my family was done in keeping with the Universal Energy. That is the difference."

"So, Master, it is possible to have wealth and be part of the Universal Energy?"

"Yes, as long as the distractions of the wealth and what it can buy do not distract you from the path to inner peace and happiness. There are many who have acquired their wealth at the expense of others. They are not truly happy for they must always worry about what they have."

"Do you worry about the wealth your family has accumulated?"

"I do not worry about it, but I do want it to be used wisely and not stolen or squandered. That is why it is in safe keeping until I return."

"Why did you give me the amulet? I could have taken it and requested the treasure."

"You don't know what the treasure is. If you received your share, it would not be with you for long and you would be back to where you originally started and that is with nothing."

"How did you know I was going to follow you and not ask the Abbot for my part once I learned about the fortune?"

"You are here now aren't you?"

"Yes, I am here now and intend to stay with you and learn." He paused, then asked. "But what is the treasure?"

"Are you happy?"

"Yes, Master, I am happy. In fact I don't think I have ever been as happy as I am with you."

"If you are happy, then don't concern yourself with the treasure."

Pei Ke smiled ruefully.

"Of course, you are right, Master. I shouldn't concern myself with something that is not mine."

As they traveled that day, Liu had Pei Ke walk in a semi-crouched position. He would take a few steps forward and then take a very quick diagonal step either to the left or right. After he did this for an hour, Liu had him walk backwards for an hour. Pei Ke knew the training was good for him, but he didn't particularly like it. As he was doing these and other walking patterns, however, he was in deep thought, which helped him to take his mind off the discomfort.

His mind returned more than once to their earlier conversation. He understood that Liu wanted to be peaceful with himself, and he did what he did to insure he was in harmony with the Universal Tao. Pei Ke understood the words, but there was this underlying feeling that life would be more enjoyable if he had money. He had always been poor, and before he'd met Liu, there had been little or no prospect his condition in life would ever change. Now there was a new prospect for him, and he still wasn't sure what to make of that.

Slowly, they drew closer to Beijing. Like their travels before, there were new things to see. For Pei Ke, it was not only the landscape but also the people. They had traveled through many different agricultural areas. In some areas there were fields of rice and in others he saw wheat growing. As always, there were the bamboo forests.

Towards the end of the day, they approached a small rural community. From a distance, it was about the same size as others they had been through. As they drew closer, however, it appeared to be deserted.

Upon reaching the center of the town, they suddenly heard a roar of distressed voices coming from the opposite side of the village. They cautiously approached and were surprised to find what appeared to be everyone in town. It was an eerie sight.

As soon as they turned the corner, they heard a horse galloping up behind them. They spun around to see a man on horseback waving them forward. His broad sword was in one hand as he held on to the reins of the horse with the other.

"Move along and get with the others," the man growled.

"We do not live here," said Liu.

"I don't care if you live here or not, move along."

"What do you want?" said Liu.

"I want you to move along. Now stop asking questions and get with the others."

"As I told you," said Liu, "we are simply passing through. We are not part of this village. Please let us pass," said Liu.

"No, you're here now," the rider spat, "so now you're part of this village. Move along or die."

He raised his broadsword as if to strike Liu and Pei Ke felt a momentary pang of sympathy for the man. He didn't know who he was dealing with.

In a blur, Liu stepped to the horse's head and touched a point on its neck. The animal reared up wildly and the rider tumbled screaming to the ground. Liu stepped forward quickly and disarmed the man.

The scuffle did not go unnoticed. Three armed men emerged from the crowd running towards Liu and Pei Ke.

"Master," Pei Ke said nervously.

"I see them."

Liu looked around to assess his position.

"Pei Ke, take this knife."

As before, Liu pulled the knife from his sleeve. Pei Ke wondered why it never fell out. It was a stupid thought and he berated himself for his lack of focus. He took the knife and his mind flashed back to the mountain weeks ago, where he had inadvertently killed one of the assailants who had attached the Liu compound.

When they had been attacked by the archer, he had been too distracted by the incoming arrows and Liu's wound to think about much more than Liu's instructions. Now, however, he stood, watching the men charging him and it was all to familiar.

"Make sure this man does not get up. Can I trust you to do this?"

"Yes, Master. I will do it."

"I am depending on you, Pei Ke." He was looking directly at his protégé, his eyes stern. "This is going to be an uneven fight and I need to know where you and this man are at all times."

"I will do it," Pei Ke said again.

To the surprise of the three charging men, Liu ran right at them. He needed to draw the fight away from Pei Ke, so he charged. The distance closed quickly. Each man was carrying a broadsword and Liu had the one he'd taken from the rider. It would be one against three.

Liu's broadsword fighting technique was derived from the techniques of the great battle-hardened General, Yue Fe. Yue Fe had trained his men in Hsing-Yi Chuan, and his troops were considered to be undefeatable. The techniques were not complex but when honed to perfection, they were devastating.

From a grassy hill overlooking the village, Chen Chang and his men watched the coming fight. It had been fortuitous that, once again, he was to meet up with Liu Bin.

His father had died at the hands of Liu Bin, and he was ashamed that he had run from the fight. Chen Chang remembered what his father had said. The land the Liu family occupied belonged to the Chen family. He didn't quite know the exact details, but he had a written declaration indicating that the lands were to be given to the Chen family for services rendered. He had been entrusted with the declaration, and he carried it now safely in his shirt. He touched his shirt to reassure himself it was still there, than he turned grimly to watch the fight below.

———————

Pei Ke held the tip of the knife at the center of the man's throat as he watched his Master fight. Any move left or right would mean instant death for the horseman who had threatened them just a few minutes earlier.

Liu wasted no time. He knew nothing of these men or their skill, but he assumed that anyone carrying a broadsword knew how to use it. The three men were evenly spaced and formed a line in front of Liu as they charged. Liu stepped to his left to take on the first man. Liu ducked the man's initial swing, than with a continuous motion, he sliced parallel to the ground at the man's leg.

Liu felt the impact and the slight resistance of the blade as it cut through the man's clothes and then into his leg. The cut wasn't deep, but was on the inside of the right leg across the femoral artery. Liu knew that unless the assailant took care of the wound immediately, he would bleed out and die. It would be a quick death, depending on the depth of the wound.

Without pausing, Liu turned to the second man, who had stepped over his comrade and was swinging his broadsword at Liu. In one continuous motion, Liu blocked the downward attack to the left, then swung his broadsword down and up catching the assailant between the legs.

The high pitched scream startled the third assailant, who turned and ran back toward the villagers, who, for their part, looked on in amazement.

Liu turned quickly to see Pei Ke kneeling next to the rider with the tip of the knife against the man's throat. Liu slowly walked in the direction of the villagers, who were now angrily yelling and screaming at someone. As he approached, they were trying to grab a burly man, who was defending himself with a broad-sword. The crowd moved aside, but surrounded the burly man as Liu entered the circle.

"Kill him," shouted someone from the crowd.

"They have come here for the last time," shouted another. "We're tired of being afraid. They've beaten us and taken our crops and money for the last time. We will no longer pay them for protection when we do not need to be protected."

"Stranger, you've done us a big favor," shouted a third.

Liu was facing the burly man, who was clearly prepared to defend himself against Liu.

"You don't seem to have many friends here," said Liu.

"This stranger will be gone and when he leaves," the man shouted to the crowd, "you'll be sorry. You'll beg to pay for my protection again."

The burly man was turning his head to emphasize his words. He was obviously distracted, so Liu stepped in with his broadsword and knocked the sword from the man's hand. Liu picked up the sword and exited the circle. The burly man didn't stand a chance. At first he fought with everything he had, but there were just too many of them to fight. The villagers beat him as he cursed them. The beating and kicking continued until the burly man was silent, but even then the villagers continued to attack him, more out of revenge than anger. Liu was certain no one could live through the beating. He walked slowly back to where Pei Ke was still holding the man at knife point.

"Master, what should I do?"

"Give me the knife."

Pei Ke slowly withdrew the knife from the man's throat. He could see an indentation where he'd nervously held the blade. As he stood up, the rider suddenly grabbed the knife and jumped to his feet.

Pei Ke was startled, but he threw his hands up to make sure he wasn't cut. The rider stabbed at Pei Ke's stomach, but Pei Ke instinctively blocked downward with his right hand as he stepped to the left. The assailant's right hand went to the right as Pei Ke controlled the knife hand. He stepped in with his left foot and kicked the man in the knee as he grabbed and threw him to the ground. He immediately followed through with a crushing blow to the man's throat.

Both Liu and Pei Ke could hear the gurgling sound as the man gasped for breath. In his last breath, and with fear in his eyes, the man coughed up blood and died. Pei Ke looked in horror at what he had just done.

"Master, I didn't mean to do that," he said in horror. "I only reacted out of fear of being hurt. You know I wouldn't purposely hurt someone. Is there something we can do for him? Did I do the right thing?"

"You did what you had to do," said Liu.

Inwardly, however, Liu thought that it would have been better not to kill the man. He wouldn't tell that to Pei Ke, who would have years of guilt to get rid of.

Liu and Pei Ke turned to see most of the villagers looking for the last man who had fled from Liu's original attack. A couple of men came over to Liu and Pei Ke.

"Stranger, you have done us a great favor. These men have been terrorizing us for over a year. Their activities were getting more violent as we protested their actions. We all are indebted to you two for what you have done for us. Please stay with us for the night and have a meal with us."

Liu looked up at the sun and then for some reason looked off into the distance. He sensed an evilness lurking in the distance. He knew they had at least three more hours of travel time, but felt it was necessary to stay with the villagers for the night. He had to admit to himself he was tired and really did need to rest.

"Thank you for your hospitality. We both are hungry and could use a rest, and we do need a place to stay for the night."

"Good, it is settled, you will stay here in the village for the night. We don't have a lot to offer, but we will make you feel at home."

Liu once again looked in the direction of the distant hill and could see men standing there. The evilness emanating from the men in the distance was similar if not identical to the evilness he had experienced on the day he had killed Chen Su. He was certain they were intent on seeing what had happened in the village. It was not a coincidence that these men were on the hill. They must have been following him since he'd left the temple. He knew there was going to be an unpleasant meeting when they finally came together, and he hoped Pei Ke would be up to the pending altercation.

He looked in the direction of Pei Ke, who seemed oblivious to the presence of the men on the hill. He still had not developed the instinct of feeling the changes in the Universal Energy. He would have to train Pei Ke a little harder on the development of internal energy and how it manifests itself in our surroundings.

Liu knew all things had energy, and the energy was like a wave that emanated from everyone and everything. This energy was the Universal Energy, but it manifested itself differently and this difference was noticeable to those who had cultivated their internal Qi.

"Master, how long are we going to stay here?"

"I don't know. Let's see what the elders have planned for us. They probably want us to stay for a while to make sure they are not attacked again."

From his location Liu turned to see the layout of the village. He wanted to know where the exits were and where most of the buildings were located. He didn't anticipate any real problem, but he wanted to be aware of his surroundings.

Once the commotion had settled down, the elders came to speak with them.

"My name is Yang," one of them said. "We all want to thank you again for what you have done for us. What brings you this way through the countryside to our humble village?"

"My name is Liu Bin and this is my student, Pei Ke. We are traveling on this road to Beijing to visit some friends. It was just by chance we arrived at your moment of need. I hope I have not caused too much of a commotion for you and the village folk."

"Of course not," said Yang. "As we indicated to you, we would like for you to stay the night. You can stay with my family. We don't have elaborate accommodations, but we do have an available room for you to stay in. Our eldest son and his wife are away visiting her parents and will not be back for another week. You must have a meal with us. Do you have any dietary restrictions?"

"We are Buddhist and do not eat meat."

"That is no problem as we also are Buddhist and many of us in this village do not eat meat. Come let me show you around the village and meet some of the other elders. I am sure they may have questions for you."

Liu was impressed with not only the village and its layout but with the friendliness of the elders. He explained more than once how he and Pei Ke had come to be there. The conversation turned to what he did, since he looked like a monk but professed not to be one. News traveled fast through the village that he was trained in acupuncture and herbal medicine. Numerous questions came up concerning whether or not acupuncture could treat certain health issues.

Liu estimated that there were about one hundred or so people residing in the village and the immediate surrounding area, and maybe another fifty residing in outlying areas. It would be a good place for a doctor to take up residence if he wanted a small group of people to serve. He consciously filed the information in the back of his head for future reference.

Seeing the peacefulness of the village, his thoughts turned to his own family. His parents had long ago passed away and he had isolated himself from his brother and the rest of his family to pursue his own agenda of being one with the Tao. Their unfortunate death, however, had left a void in his heart.

His decision to go to Beijing might not have been the best choice. However, for some unexplained reason, he was compelled to go there. Maybe he would be able to explain this need to go when he arrived. He knew a few people in Beijing, and he really wanted to visit with them one last time. He had not seen his friends for a number of years. Some of his friends were martial artists like himself and others were in the healing arts.

As a student, he had studied with them for varying degrees of time. They had all gone their own way in life, and he wanted to find out how they were using their healing skills. He also knew that some who had trained in martial arts by now would be teaching on their own and probably had many students. Some of them who had been studying medicine worked in the local hospital or had a private practice of their own.

Liu's thoughts turned to Pei Ke. It would be good for him to have a little practice in the village while they were there. He thought that maybe they should stay for a couple of days.

Liu turned to Yang.

"I noticed there were some men on the hill to the west of us. Is there any reason you can think of why someone would be interested in what is taking place here in the village?"

Yang immediately turned to look at the hill Liu was referring to but he could see no one.

"There is no one on the hill."

"Yes, whoever was there has gone for now. However, it doesn't mean they won't come back. Does someone live on the hill?"

"No one," said Yang. "Do you know who these people are?"

"No. You should have someone in the village make some inquiries about any strangers in the area. It might be part of the same group harassing you."

"I will have some of the younger men see what they can find out. Should they be looking for anything in particular?"

"They should be looking for anything out of the ordinary or out of place. If the people I spotted do not belong here, they will need to stay somewhere. Maybe you could have the men contact people in the outlying area and see if these men are camping out. You don't want to be caught by surprise during the night."

"That's a good idea. Now let me take you to my home and you can wait there for me until I return."

"For now, I will stay here in the center of the village and watch and see what is happening. Is that all right with you?"

"Of course," said Yang. "I will be back shortly."

———————

Chen Chang had witnessed the altercation in the village from his vantage point on the hill. He couldn't see the faces of the two men who won the fight, but from what he observed, he was positive it was Liu Bin and his young student. Few people could move as quickly and with such expertise, especially against weapons. He remembered the time he'd gone up against Liu. He felt his arm where Liu had cut him. The wound had been deep. He didn't have full use of his arm yet, but he could see and feel improvement each day.

He was lucky to have escaped with his life, and he knew it. Liu had killed his father weeks before, and now he was going to avenge his father's death. He again touched the small scroll in his shirt. It was proof that the Chen family was the rightful owners of the land. He smiled grimly.

# Chapter Twenty-three

Mr. Yang returned shortly and motioned for Liu and Pei Ke to follow him.

"I know this is quite abrupt on my part, but if you are a doctor would you mind seeing this elderly person. She does not feel well and maybe you can help her.

"Of course," said Liu. "Just lead the way."

The three of them walked across the village grounds and Mr. Yang knocked on the door of a nondescript house. The door opened and Yang introduced Liu and Pei Ke to Mrs. Lo.

"Come in," said Mrs. Lo.

Liu, Pei Ke and Mr. Yang walked into a small but nicely decorated home. From the way the altar at the far end of the room was placed and the scrolls on the wall, Liu knew that the woman was quite religious.

"I understand you helped with those nasty bandits who keep coming to take our money and crops."

"It is fortunate we came through your village when we did."

"The gods must have looked down favorably on us and our plight," said the woman.

"Mr. Yang said you do not feel well. I am a doctor. This is my student, Pei Ke. Together we will try to help you. What is the problem?"

"For some reason I've been afflicted with pain, soreness, and swelling of the joints in my legs and arms. Sometimes the pain is worse than others. When it's severe, I have limited range of motion. Is this something you know how to treat?"

"I have successfully treated this type of problem before. We need to know more information before we can treat you. I am going to ask you some questions; but before I do, I want Pei Ke to ask you some questions of his own."

Pei Ke was momentarily caught off guard by Liu's request, but he quickly recovered from his momentary surprise. He had done this before and he was confident he could discern some valuable information about Mrs. Lo. As Liu watched and listened, Pei Ke went through the four basic diagnostic methods of inspection, listening and smelling, inquiring, and palpitation. When he was finished, he turned to Liu who continued the line of questioning.

"Mrs. Lo, from what you have told us already we can assume you have had this problem for some time."

"Yes, and it can be quite painful. Sometimes it is in my fingers and sometimes it is in my shoulders. In fact, from day to day and even during the same day, it moves around my body from one area to another."

"It is called a Bi Syndrome," said Liu. "These syndromes are characterized by a blockage of the vital energy and blood in the meridian system of your body."

"What causes this problem?" asked Mrs. Lo.

"It sometimes affects people living in cold, damp, and windy areas. The ancient people believe that these environmental factors of wind, cold, and dampness enter into the body from the outside. Many times this problem becomes worse when there is a sudden change of weather from warm to cold or dry to wet. When the problem is severe, the patient has pain and swelling in the joints. Often the patient has difficulty moving his or her fingers and toes. I have even seen cases so advanced that the joints become deformed to the point where the patient has difficulty walking.

"Mrs. Lo, I need to feel your pulses to differentiate your problem."

Liu felt the pulses on the radial artery. Pei Ke mentally went through the process of taking the pulses as he watched Liu perform one of the most delicate of diagnostic protocols.

"Pei Ke, I want you to feel her pulses and tell me what you find."

Pei Ke moved next to Mrs. Lo. He could tell she was watching him very intently to see if he did exactly as Liu had done. After a couple of minutes Pei Ke let go of Mrs. Lo's wrist and looked at Liu.

"Well, what have you discovered?" asked Liu.

Quite hesitantly Pei Ke said. "Her pulses are superficial and slow."

"Good," said Liu.

"Now I want you to look at her tongue and tell me what you see."

Mrs. Lo opened her mouth and stuck her tongue out so Liu and Pei Ke could analyze the shape, coating, and color of the tongue.

"Master, her tongue has a thin white sticky coating."

"From seeing the tongue would you guess she has an excess or a deficiency?"

"Master, she has a deficiency."

"Why do you say that?"

"If she had an excess, the tongue would probably have a yellow coating."

"Good," said Liu

"Mrs. Lo, there are a number of different Bi syndromes in Chinese medicine. As I indicated before, a Bi syndrome is caused by wind, cold, and dampness entering into the meridian system of the body. It is also due to an overall weakness of the body with a deficiency of Yang energy. The weakness allows the cold, dampness, and wind to enter the body through the pores.

"There is Painful Bi Syndrome, Fixed Bi Syndrome, Wandering Bi Syndrome, and Heat Bi Syndrome. Painful Bi Syndrome is characterized by the patient complaining of severe stabbing pain in one or more joints. Usually the pain is helped by the application of heat from a moxa stick. If you felt the joint, you probably would not feel any heat in the joint, and since there was no heat there wouldn't be any redness. The tongue coating would be thin and white, and the pulse would be taut and tense.

"When you analyze this situation, it is readily evident that the cold has caused the slowing of the Qi in the meridians. The lack of Qi flowing to the joints in time causes the joints to be painful and stiff. The application of heat feels good to the patient and gives the patient some relief. A white coating on the tongue is indicative of a deficiency in the body. A tense pulse is indicative of a coldness affecting the body."

"Master Liu, my symptoms are similar to what you just described, but not quite the same."

"Yes, I know. Let me finish with the other possible Bi Syndromes. This information may be boring for you, but it is helpful to Pei Ke.

"Yes, go on," said Mrs. Lo. "It's not boring. It gives me confidence in your abilities."

Liu smiled and continued where he left off.

"A Fixed Bi Syndrome is characterized by a feeling of numbness in the joints. There is also the feeling of heaviness in the limbs. The pain becomes more pronounced on days when there is cold, wind, or dampness. The tongue has a white sticky coating, and there is generally a soft pulse.

"A Heat Bi Syndrome is characterized by pain and swelling in one or more joints. The pain is severe, causing restricted motion. The patient often complains of thirst. The tongue has a yellow coating on it. The pulse is rolling and rapid.

"When you look at the symptoms, the heat is consistent with the yellowish tongue. The reason there is heat is because the wind, cold, and dampness Bi syndromes have been in the body for an extended period of time and have turned into heat.

"A Wandering Bi Syndrome is characterized by pain in the wrists, knees, ankles, or elbows, causing limited range of motion due to the pain. Sometimes the patient complains of chills and fever. The tongue usually has a thin and sticky coating, and the pulse is usually superficial and slow. Quite often, the patient will not only complain of having pain that seems to wander through the body but also of chills and fever."

"Master, based on what you've said, that is what I have. How do I get rid of it?"

"Depending on which of the four Bi Syndromes you experience, it is treated in different ways. Since there is wind, cold, and dampness in the meridian system, we need to choose acupuncture points designed to rid the body of these symptoms. Ashi points can be used in the area where there is pain. In addition, local and or distal points associated with the meridians being affected can be used.

"In general, when there is Fixed Bi the best way to treat it is with acupuncture and moxibustion. For Painful Bi, the needles usually are inserted deeper and kept in place for a longer period of time. When the diagnosis is Wandering Bi, it is important to use one of the many reducing methods to solve the problem. For Heat Bi the reducing method would also be used.

"Since you have Wandering Bi, we are going to use the reduction method of acupuncture to solve the problem. Where do you have the majority of pain at this moment?"

"Master, the majority of my pain is in my wrists."

"Pei Ke, one of the most important points for eliminating a wind condition in the body is Feng Chi. I also use this point when I am treating someone who has a common cold. It is very effective, and the patient will usually see immediate relief for the cold symptoms.

"Since she has pain in her wrists, I am also going to use Ashi Points and local points.

"Mrs. Lo, may I do some acupuncture on you today?"

"Yes, of course. Are you going to do the acupuncture or is your student going to do it?"

"I will do it. Pei Ke, please get my needles out of the sack and make sure they are clean and sterile."

Pei Ke did as he was told as Liu continued to talk with Mrs. Lo. When Pei Ke was done, he gave the needles to Liu.

"Pei Ke, I want you to watch what I am doing. You can ask questions when I have all these needles in place," said Liu.

Pei Ke watched as Liu began inserting the needles into Mrs. Lo. He first inserted a needle into the Feng Chi point on the left side and then another on the right side. He continued inserting needles into Ashi, local, and distal points. Pei Ke saw him using points he had never seen him use before and made a mental note to ask him about those points.

When Liu had finished putting in the needles he turned to Pei Ke and nodded for him to ask questions.

"Master I know some of those points from other patients you have treated, but there are some I have never seen you use before."

"To which points are you referring?" asked Liu.

Pei Ke pointed to three separate points. Liu nodded.

"Before I explain these other points I want to give you some information on the Feng Chi Point. It is classically known that wind can enter the body through this point and block the flow of energy in the body. When you insert a needle into this point, the wind is dispersed and the energy can flow correctly. This point not only disperses wind, which is an external condition, but it also dispels wind which has become internal. This point can be used to treat headaches, dizziness, neck pain, common cold, and the flu.

"Basically, this point is used to treat a myriad of problems related to the head, neck, eyes, ears, and shoulders. Pei Ke you need to remember the importance of this point. This is one of those points you do not want to forget."

Liu went on to describe in detail the other points he used and the logic behind why he chose those points. Twenty minutes later Liu took the needles out.

"How do you feel now, Mrs. Lo?"

Mrs. Lo moved both of her wrists. She looked at her wrists and hands to see if she could detect a difference.

"The pain is much better, but it is not totally gone. There seems to be less stiffness and swelling in the wrists. Do I need more treatments?"

"Yes, it would be appropriate for you to have a series of treatments to really help this condition. I will do another treatment on you tomorrow and it should help you even more with the pain."

"Thank you very much," said Mrs. Lo. "How can I ever repay you for what you have done?"

"Mrs. Lo, I want you to rest here for the remainder of the day. You may feel sleepy later on. If so, just go to bed and don't worry about things you have to do. I understand there are others in the village I can see and the day is still young for me to do some good."

Liu and Pei Ke left Mrs. Lo and went outside. Mr. Yang who brought them to Mrs. Lo's was waiting for them.

"I asked some of the younger men to explore the hill as you requested, but they could not find anything or anyone up there. Are you sure you saw someone there?"

"Maybe I was mistaken," said Liu.

"Master, there is someone else I would like for you to see if you don't mind. He has been a friend for many years and is one of the elders of this village. You saw him briefly but you were not formally introduced to him."

"Take me to him, and maybe I can help him."

Liu, Pei Ke, and Mr. Yang walked across the open village to a house that was smaller than most of the other houses. Yang knocked on the door and a rather thin, elderly man answered the door.

"This is Mr. Po," said the gentleman.

Liu and Pei Ke bowed and introduced themselves.

"Come in," said Mr. Po. "I understand you are a doctor."

"Yes, I have been trained in acupuncture and Chinese herbal formulas."

"We used to have a doctor here a few years ago, but one day he just disappeared. We have been looking for someone to replace him for quite some time. We are not a large community, but we do have many who come to the village from outlying areas. There isn't any large town or village for many miles and this place, while it is very small, is the hub of activity for this area. You might want to consider staying here. We can let you use one of our vacant buildings, and we can provide you with food. Give it some thought before you say no."

"Thank you," said Liu. "I will consider it."

Pei Ke looked at Liu in surprise, wondering whether his master was being serious or simply polite. There was nothing here for Liu or him.

"Now that I am here with you, what can I help you with today?"

"I have bad insomnia. Sometimes I do not fall asleep until the middle of the night and if I do fall asleep, I cannot stay asleep. Is there something you can do to help me?"

"Pei Ke is one of my students, and he is going to ask you a series of questions. Try to answer the questions as best you can. There is a reason for each question, even if they don't seem appropriate to your condition."

Pei Ke was pleased that Liu had asked him to do this again. He knew the more he was involved in the process, the more he would learn. It was better for him to be involved early with patients than later on. Study and book learning was good, but it was no substitute for actually dealing with a patient one-on-one.

Pei Ke started out with the four basic diagnostic questions. This time, he went more in depth than he had done with Mrs. Lo. He truly wanted to discover the essence of why Mr. Po had his insomnia. As he inquired about the patients personal background, family background, and social background he saw Liu nodding his approval.

Pei Ke looked at Mr. Po's tongue and took note of its size, shape, and color. He also observed the color and texture of the coating on the tongue and checked to see if there were markings on it. It would be one clue for him to tell his master what was wrong with Mr. Po.

He also noted the color of the patient's skin, along with the texture of the skin. He observed the hands and finger nails to see if there was anything unusual. He looked at the face to see if he could discern anything that would give him further clues to the cause of the insomnia.

When Pei Ke was done with his examination and questions he turned to Liu for approval.

"Mr. Po, how old are you?" asked Liu.

Instantly Pei Ke admonished himself for not asking the question. It was a simple question, and he made a mental note to ask it in the future. He also remembered that he should have asked Po what type of work he did. Stress had a lot to do with the balance of energy in the body. Too much mental stress affects the heart which, in turn, affects the mind.

"I am sixty-five," said Mr. Po.

"What is your diet like? What foods do you commonly eat?" asked Liu?

"I don't like rice too much, but I really like to eat noodles. I have noodles at almost every meal," said Mr. Po. "I am Buddhist, so I don't eat meat, but I eat some vegetables every day with the noodles."

"When do you eat your last meal of the day?" asked Liu. "Maybe I should ask how often do you eat?"

"I have breakfast, lunch, and dinner, along with a large snack just before bedtime."

"How often do you follow this routine?" asked Liu.

"Every day," said Po.

Pei Ke again admonished himself for not asking the questions. He was sure the line of questions Liu was formulating had something to do with the insomnia. *How did he know to ask those specific questions? It must have come from prior experience*, thought Pei Ke.

"Mr. Po, part of our diagnostic process is to take your pulses. Your pulses will tell us where the energy is blocked in your body. I would like for Pei Ke to take your pulses."

"Of course," said Po.

Liu gave Pei Ke an approving nod, and Pei Ke sat down next to Mr. Po while Liu observed. Pei Ke made sure Po's wrists were placed approximately at heart level on the table and supported appropriately. He debated for a few seconds as to which side to do first, but concluded that it really didn't matter since he was going to do both sides.

He placed his middle finger first on the middle pulse as he had previously been instructed by Liu. He felt the pulses at the required depths and made a mental note of what he had found. He continued to do this for all the pulses on both wrists. When he was done he asked Mr. Po a series of questions. He turned to Liu, waiting for further instructions.

"Mr. Po," said Liu. "I am going to also feel your pulses to see where the imbalance of energy exists."

Liu did the same as Pei Ke, with one significant distinction. He took more time than Pei Ke with each position as though he was making some distinction between the pulses. After a few minutes, which seemed like an eternity, Liu turned to Pei Ke.

"What did you discover from the pulses?"

"Master, the heart pulse was weak."

"What does that tell you?"

"Since it is not full, it must be deficient."

"Good. What else did you discover?"

"You mean about the pulse?"

"Not only the pulses. Everything from your differential diagnosis."

"When I asked him about his insomnia, he indicated he had problems falling asleep. When he did fall asleep, his sleep was disturbed by vivid dreams. He indicated that he'd had a poor memory for the last couple of years. His energy was not so good and many times he felt tired and just didn't want to do anything. He forced himself to do things, however, because he was one of the elders of the village and others depended on his council and actions."

"When you looked at him what did you find?"

"He's thin. Everyone in the village is thin, but I think he is thinner than the rest of them. I never thought of that as a clue or possible problem."

"You asked him about his urination, bowels, and other things. You did good, but you forgot to ask him about his heart."

Pei Ke looked at Liu and then at Mr. Po, and then again back at Liu.

"Do you have any heart problems we should know about?" asked Liu.

"My heart flutters sometimes. I can feel it during the day and also sometimes when I try to go to sleep. I feel my heart beating."

*That has to be a major clue in this diagnostic process,* thought Pei Ke. I missed it, and it is probably one of the major indications.

"Pei Ke, what did you notice about his tongue?"

"It is pale, but other than that, I didn't notice anything unusual. There were no strange markings, and the shape and length seemed to be normal."

Liu turn to Mr. Po.

"Mr. Po, insomnia can be caused by a number of different things. We can classify them as dysfunctions, disharmony, upward disturbances, and deficiencies. To treat you effectively, we need to isolate the many factors causing each one of these conditions.

"If you had an unsatisfactory balance or disharmony between your heart and kidney, then you would probably have symptoms such as dizziness, ringing in the ears, low back pain, and a burning sensation in your palms and the soles of your feet. I would expect your pulses to be thready and somewhat rapid. I would expect not to see a pale tongue, but rather a red tongue somewhat redder than normal. You don't have these signs and symptoms so my analysis is that you do not have a disharmony between your heart and kidney Qi.

"If you indicated that throughout the day and evening you felt anxious or fearful and had frequent headaches along with a bitter taste in your mouth, I would expect you to have a pulse that was quite taut. However, you don't indicate this to us, and on examination we find your pulses were not taut. This eliminates the possibility of a disturbance of Liver Fire Rising.

"If you'd said you belched quite often and had discomfort in the middle of your chest below the sternum, and had problems with your bowels I would suspect your tongue would have a sticky coating to it. When Pei Ke looked at your tongue, however, you did not have that type of coating. I would also expect you to have a rolling pulse, which you did not. Therefore, I would eliminate the possibility of there being some sort of dysfunction of the stomach.

"Instead, you indicated that you had difficulty falling asleep and your sleep was fitful with dreams. You said you felt listless and that you had heart palpitations. And Pei Ke saw a thin coating on your tongue. Since there was a thin coating on the tongue, I would suspect a weak pulse, which you heard Pei Ke say you had."

"Yes. That's exactly what I have," said Mr. Po. "What is wrong with me?"

"I suspect you have a condition we refer to as a deficiency of heart Qi and spleen Qi."

"What causes that?" asked Po.

"There can be a number of different causes. In your case, I suspect there are two reasons for this problem. First, you have a one-sided diet eating too many noodles and eating them too late in the evening. The stomach is responsible for receiving and processing the food we eat. After the food is processed, it is sent to the spleen.

"The main function of the spleen is the manufacture of Qi and Blood. There are not enough nutrients in your food to support your blood. You do not get enough circulation to your heart and your head. Your diet has interrupted the normal function of this organ. That is why you have palpitations and poor memory, and are tired and weak. The spleen has an influence on the heart, which is the seat of our emotions and has a direct influence on our mind.

"The second factor is the stress you are experiencing by being one of the elders of this village. We all react to stress in different ways. What is stressful for one person is not stressful for another. We have to evaluate the stress in the context of the person and his or her station in life."

"Can you treat me for this problem?" asked Po.

"Yes, this problem can be treated with acupuncture. But you must also change your diet and realize that stress is one factor in this problem. Would you like for me to treat you now?"

"Yes, please," said Po.

"Pei Ke, get the needles ready for me."

"Yes, Master."

As Po was making himself comfortable on the bed, Pei Ke was finishing up with the preparation of the needles.

"Pei Ke, the first acupuncture point I am going to use is Shen Men. It is one of the major acupuncture points on the Heart Meridian. Its name literally means 'Spirit Gate.' As the name suggests, it has a positive effect on your mind. It is traditionally used to treat insomnia, sadness, fear, uncontrolled hysteria, and any type of heart problems. This point is exceptional for its ability to calm the mind and the spirit. It is one of those points you should consider any time you suspect there is an emotional component to your diagnosis.

"It can also be used in conjunction with a wide range of other points to solve very specific health care issues.

"Mr. Po, are you ready?"

"Yes," said Po.

"Pei Ke, I want you to watch closely how I do this treatment."

Pei Ke watched intently as Liu inserted a needle into the Shen Men point on the left side and then on the opposite side. He continued inserting other needles into selected points. When he was done, he turned to Po.

"How do you feel?"

"Very relaxed and peaceful. It feels like a burden has been taken off my shoulders and my mind feels clearer. It's a nice feeling; I hope it lasts for a long time."

"Pei Ke, do you have any questions?"

"No, Master. I have learned a lot from watching you today. Allowing me to play a greater role in treating patients has really helped. I will follow more closely with your technique in diagnosis and try to remember to ask questions."

As they were finishing the treatment with Mr. Po, the door opened and a woman in her mid-forties came in with three girls trailing behind her.

"This is my wife and my three daughters," said Po. The wife and the young girls all bowed in unison to Liu and Pei Ke. Pei Ke judged the oldest daughter to be about his age and the other two were about two years apart. The wife was much younger than Mr. Po, so Pei Ke guessed he'd either had an earlier wife or had more than one. This was a large family for so small a house. They must all sleep in the same room. He'd only seen a couple of rooms when they'd entered. Maybe they had adjoining rooms he couldn't see.

As he looked at the oldest girl, his mind immediately went to Mei Li and Hua Yee. He missed them both and wished he could be with them or they could be with him. He knew it was wishful thinking. He was going to be with one or the other. He thought of the conversations he'd had with both of them and of their appealing attributes. He couldn't make up his mind which one was more beautiful and he could see advantages to being with each of them. If he married Mei Li, he knew he could continue his martial arts training under her father Wei Ken De. If he married Hua Yee, he would have access to the Liu ancestral lands and fortune. It was really a dilemma and he did not know how to get around it. He knew Liu suspected he was in a dilemma, but in this case, he didn't want to ask Liu for his advice.

He wanted to go with Liu to Beijing, but he also wanted to return to see both of the young ladies he had left. When he had departed, he was sure there had been a mutual feeling between each of them. Of course, there was no way for him to be sure, but he still felt an urgency to make a decision about them one way or the other. Wei Ken De could easily marry off Mei Li any time there appeared a suitable suitor. Although Mei Li would have some say in the matter, her father would have the final say.

On the other hand, if there was a suitor for Hua Yee, it would be appropriate for Mr. Wu, who was looking after Hua Yee, to wait for Liu to return to the family village.

"Pei Ke."

Pei Ke was pulled out of his thoughts to see Liu looking at him.

"Is there anything you want to ask of Mr. Po before we depart?"

"No, Master."

Throughout the early evening they treated a few more people. Word had spread quickly through the village about the stranger who had spared them from the crooks, who also happened to be a doctor. He and his young assistant were willing to help anyone who asked.

Everyone wanted to put them up for the night. There were many offers, but Liu explained they were very simple people and did not need or want for much. The villagers, however, would have none of it and insisted they be treated with a good meal and the best sleeping quarters in the village.

# CHAPTER TWENTY-FOUR

The following morning Pei Ke and Liu arose early to practice Qi Gong. At first, they were by themselves as the early morning sun rose in the east, but it wasn't more than a few minutes before some of the villagers came out of their houses and found Liu and Pei Ke practicing. A crowd soon developed as the two martial artists went through their routines.

When they had finished, everyone started asking questions. Liu tried to answer them to the best of his ability. Soon they were asking Pei Ke as many questions as they were asking Liu. Pei Ke explained briefly where they had come from and where they were going. As the two of them were answering questions, Mr. Po pushed to the front of the now expanding group of villagers.

"Master Liu," he shouted. The volume of his voice surprised the villagers, for it was out of character for him to be so loud.

"Many of you have heard me complain of my insomnia. Yesterday in the late afternoon, Master Liu treated me with acupuncture. Well, last night I fell asleep immediately and did not wake up till early this morning. I feel rested. More rested than I have felt in years. You are truly a miracle worker. You must stay with us and be part of our village."

"I agree," said Mrs. Lo, who had pushed her way to the center of the group.

"Yesterday, I was also treated by Master Liu for pain in my wrist. It isn't completely gone, but it feels better than it has in a long time. You definitely need to stay here and be part of what we have to offer."

Others who Liu had treated the day before joined in urging him to stay. Pei Ke was overwhelmed with what he saw. These people were willing to accept Liu immediately because of what he could do with just a few needles.

Liu raised his hands for everyone to be quiet. He looked around the group and nodded to those he had treated.

"Thank you for your generosity, but we must be on our way today. But before we leave, I would like to see those I saw yesterday and give them another treatment."

Liu could hear groans from the group of people. He knew they wanted him to stay but he needed to be on his way. Liu visited with Mrs. Lo, Mr. Po, and the others he had treated the night before. It was mid-morning when he finished with the last of the patients. He said his good-byes to the last patient and walked out the door. To his surprise there was an enormous group of people in front of the door blocking the way. In unison, they all clapped and bowed down to Liu and Pei Ke.

Liu did not know what to do. He was accustomed to people giving him thanks for the healing, but he had never had a situation like this where a whole village and possibly some living outside the village were giving thanks for the little he did.

"Come Master Liu," said one of the elders. "We want you to see something."

The group surrounded Liu and Pei Ke and walked with them down the street. There were some women in the door-ways of some of the houses holding on to the little children. They bowed as Liu and Pei Ke passed.

Pei Ke had never seen anything like this before. They were treating Liu almost as if he was a prince. They were even trying to touch him, and in the process they were touching Pei Ke. For Pei Ke, it was a wonderful feeling to have so many people pay respect, even if he knew he'd done less than Liu. He recognized that this was truly a deep respect, and not the mandatory respect one has to pay to the royal family.

Pei Ke could see Liu was feeling good about what was happening. Liu did not often smile, but there was more than just a hint of a smile on his face.

Everyone was talking to him at the same time and he didn't know who to answer first. Some were even talking to Pei Ke who tried to answer questions.

At the far end of the village, the group with Liu and Pei Ke in the middle arrived at a modest house that even had windows. Part of the group separated so Liu and Pei Ke were in front of the main door. One of the elders opened the door and gestured for Liu and Pei Ke to enter.

"A year or so ago we had a doctor," said one of the elders. "He was called to another village on an emergency case. He never arrived at the other village. We don't know what happened to him. It was strange, but shortly after his disappearance those thugs arrived. We suspected there was a connection, but there was nothing we could prove.

"This is the house we let him use. We suspect foul play, because all of his things are still in his house just where he left them when he hurried off. His clothes are even here. We packed everything up neatly in case he returned. He was not married so there was no one but him.

"Now, we want you to stay with us. Please use this house. We will also try to provide you with whatever else you might need. We do not have a lot but we are self sufficient and can take care of ourselves."

Liu looked through the door. Pei Ke saw him turn and look up to the hill far off into the distance. Pei Ke followed his line of sight and looked at the hill as well. There was nothing there. As Liu looked, he did not sense any evilness. All he sensed was peacefulness and happiness in the surrounding area.

He looked at Pei Ke and saw a slight smile on his student's face. Liu looked out over the crowd. Off to one side, he could see a young woman with a child cuddled in her arms. The baby was crying softly as the mother held him tight to her bosom. He could just see the top of the infant's head. What he saw puzzled him for a minute. After a second glance, he realized what was wrong with the child.

*The child needs help and needs it soon*, thought Liu. If I leave, the child is going to suffer.

As Liu scanned the villagers, he could see most of them were healthy, but there were some who really needed assistance. Unless there was a doctor in the village soon, some of these people would become worse. He knew he could help if he had the time to devote to their care.

"We are committed to going to Beijing," he said finally. "But we can stay for a couple of days."

There was a loud cheer from the villagers. The elder nudged Liu and Pei Ke through the door. It was dark inside and had a faint musty smell. Someone opened the windows and the combination of light from the door and the light from the windows helped them to adjust their eyes to the surroundings.

They were standing in what appeared to be an outer parlor. He was sure this made do as a doctor's office. There was a sturdy wooden table where the doctor must have sat. There were chairs on both sides of the table and obviously the doctor had his patients sit with him as he visited with them.

Benches lined one wall where others could sit. It was a strange custom, but when someone became sick and went to the doctor it was not unusual for the whole family, including grandparents to go as well. The whole family thus was made part of the healing process.

Along the side of one wall, there was a cabinet with maybe a hundred or so small drawers. The writing on some of the drawers was faded, but the ones he could see reminded him of an herbal store. The doctor must have had a generous supply of herbs to take care of the villagers. His quick scan of the names on the drawers confirmed that the most important herbs in Chinese Medicine were here. Or were they?

Liu walked over to the wall and opened one of the drawers. Yes, there were herbs in the draw. He opened others and found they also contained herbs. He would have to check the others later to make sure there was enough to take care of the basic health issues of the villagers.

"There are other rooms in the back," said the elder who had opened the door. "There are two bedrooms and a kitchen. They are not big, but it can accommodate the two of you while you are here. We had anticipated the previous doctor would one day get married and have a family so we tried to make this as hospitable as possible." He sighed.

"He was a good doctor. He looked after us and the surrounding area including some of the other villages."

"What was his name?" asked Liu.

"His name was Pao. He came from the south. He mentioned where he learned his skill, but I have forgotten the place. It wasn't anyplace we had heard of. We are not very worldly here; we are common folk, but are honest and kind. We miss him, but welcome you to stay here and lead a peaceful life with us."

"Thank you," said Liu. "I must say again we are only going to be here for a short time before we must move on."

Pei Ke noted the difference between what Liu had said a few minutes ago about staying only a couple of days and what he had just said about staying for only a short time. Maybe Liu liked this place, and maybe he would want to stay here. As he thought about it, he dismissed the idea. If Liu wanted to stay anyplace, he would definitely choose his ancestral house. Everything he wanted was there including the peacefulness he cherished.

The village elder went outside. Seconds later, there was a roar of approval from the villagers. Liu once again smiled. The elder poked his head through one of the open windows.

"A woman from the village will be arriving in a few minutes to air out this place and clean it up for you."

Liu looked at the contents of the herbal cabinet as Pei Ke looked at the books on one of the shelves. He saw the basic writings of acupuncture and herbal medicine along with writings from Confucius, Lao Tze, and others. He picked up one of the books and began to read. He really wanted the book. It explained many aspects of Chinese Medicine similar to what Liu had told him, but in a different context. After a few minutes there was a knock on the door and Pei Ke went to open it.

As he opened the door he saw three women, each with a girl about Pei Ke's age by their side. Each girl cast her eyes downward. The women and girls all bowed in unison, and Pei Ke returned the bow.

"We are here to clean the house for you," said one of the women. "The house has been closed for some time, and we want it to be presentable for you during your stay with us. If you would let us come in, we can all get started."

Pei Ke distinctly remembered the elder saying that one woman would come to clean the house, not six, but he moved aside and the women and girls entered. Liu had heard the conversation and bowed politely. The girls giggled as they bowed in respect. The women and girls immediately went to the back room. Pei Ke walked over to Liu and whispered to Liu.

"Master," he said blushing a bit, "I think these women have brought their daughters here for me to look at them."

"Yes, I know," said Liu. "It was very obvious. In most outlying villages, there is not a very large population of eligible men to choose from. Sometimes families look to other villages. Here, it is my guess there are not very many men who are as unique and interesting as you are. You are prime for them. You are handsome, intelligent, and strong—all the attributes a mother would want for her daughter."

Liu could see Pei Ke was about to panic.

"You feel trapped in this situation?" asked Liu.

"Not trapped, Master, but what am I supposed to do?" asked Pei Ke. "We are going to be here for a few days and I have no interest in these girls. I would never want to live here. I don't mean that as an insult, Master. It is certainly nice, but there is nothing here for me."

"The people in this village are willing to provide all the basic needs for any qualified doctor who wants to live here. Whoever lives here would have status. The villagers would always look up to him. Actually, I think that is why the previous doctor disappeared. Someone wanted him out of the way so they could have influence over the village."

"It's just that I have other plans," said Pei Ke.

"And what are these plans?" asked Liu.

"Foremost, I want to study with you."

"Perhaps doing nothing is the appropriate thing to do."

"Master, what have you done in similar situations?"

"Pei Ke, I have seldom been in similar situations so I cannot answer the question."

"Should I say something to the women or the girls? I don't want to mislead them. They need to understand we are doctors and we are going to leave for Beijing in a couple of days."

Liu found it interesting that Pei Ke had started to think of himself as a doctor. He thought it emphasized Pei Ke's desire to learn.

*Now what if he would just start thinking of himself as a martial artist,* Liu thought. *He knows he can do things in medicine. He now needs to know he can do things in martial arts. Time will tell.*

# CHAPTER TWENTY-FIVE

For the rest of the day, Liu and Pei Ke became acquainted with the elders and villagers. Liu made it a point to go to as many houses as possible and inquire about their health. He found the interior of the homes to be mainly the same. The village wasn't rich nor was it excessively poor. Almost everyone had about the same things: a small outer room, small kitchen, and one or more bedrooms depending on how many there were in the family.

What he did find interesting was the fact that there were not many children in each family. Most families had as many children as possible so the children could take care of the parents when the parents were old. There were just as many girls as there were boys in the general population. Of course, a boy would be more important, since the girls would leave the village and go to another family.

Liu did not spend much time with them, but of course, each one wanted to tell him a long story. He artfully indicated to each that he only had a few minutes, but in the morning after his early morning exercise, to which they could come if they wanted, he would be willing to see the villagers about their health care issues.

The conversations with the villagers were tiring but informative. He learned many things about the village which might be useful later on, when he traveled back through the village. When he had finished, he and Pei Ke returned to their assigned house.

"Pei Ke, there are two bedrooms. They are quite small but they are adequate for each of us. You can take the one on the right and I will stay in the other. The stove will keep us warm and there are plenty of blankets.

"The people in this village are very simple in their ways. Because they are simple, they are pure of spirit and without greed and envy. Because of their nature, they are very vulnerable to what other people say and do. It would be very easy to take advantage of the villagers. When we leave, I want to be able to think the village and everyone in it is just as pure and innocent as when we initially arrived. Do you understand what I am telling you?"

"Yes, Master. I fully understand and agree with what you have said."

———————

During the night, the wind blew out of the north and a couple of inches of snow fell. A fire had been lit for them and even though they could feel the coldness in the air, Pei Ke and Liu were warm under their respective blankets.

As Liu was falling asleep, his thoughts turned to this village they had entered. Was there a universal reason they were there in the village at this particular time? He would have to consult the I-Ching to find out.

Seconds before he fell asleep, a wave of unsettled energy swept through his mind. He sat up straight in his bed and looked around the tiny room. There was no one in the room, but he knew the Universal Tao had told him to be careful. Just as soon as it came, it departed. Liu put his head on the tea scented pillow and fell asleep. It would not happen tonight.

———————

At the same time that Liu was settling in for the night, Chen Chang and his men were settling in for the night in the camp they had established not far from the village. They had been in hiding ever since they saw the villagers looking for them. He knew Liu was in the village. Chen Chang's goal was to make his next attack the final attack. He didn't want to have to fight with Liu over and over again. Chen debated whether or not he should attack the village that night. The more he thought about Liu, the angrier he became. Reason won out over emotion and he decided to wait. For now.

# CHAPTER TWENTY-SIX

The next morning Liu woke up earlier than usual. He looked in on Pei Ke and found him to be sound asleep. He went to the front sitting area and looked out one of the two windows to see snow on the ground. The sky was clear and he looked at the visible glow in the east, heralding the arrival of the morning sun as it worked its way up to the horizon.

A quick glance at the ground and the undisturbed snow confirmed the village had been peaceful during the night. He knew the snow had started to fall just before he'd gone to sleep. He had not heard the sound of geese or dogs, so there were no strangers within hearing or smelling range.

It was going to be a very busy day for him. He needed to get as much energy as possible to prepare himself for what lay ahead. Pei Ke and the villagers were asleep and probably would be asleep for another hour. It was the perfect time to do his meditation.

Those wonderful ladies who had cleaned the place made a point of telling Liu and Pei Ke that a container of green tea was available, and they made sure there was enough fresh water for them to make tea in the morning. Just before retiring, Liu had started a small fire in the stove. A slight glow suggested the embers were still hot. Liu placed a little kindling on the embers and some dry grass. It immediately caught fire and soon there were enough flames to ignite the kindling and Liu had his morning fire going to heat up the little house and make his morning tea.

As the water was heating, Liu started walking around the small area of the outer room. He walked to awaken his muscles. He learned at a young age, when he first started practicing martial arts, that the body and muscles needed to be awakened from their sleep. Walking was a good way to do it. As he walked he moved his waist, shoulders, and arms. Gradually, the slight stiffness left his body.

The water came to a boil, and he poured it into the cup of fresh tea leaves. He watched as the water swirled around the leaves and they settled to the bottom of the cup. He took the cup and walked over to the table where he put the cup on the edge of the table. He sat in the chair and began his warm-up routine.

He had been practicing Qi Gong for many years and found the Qi Gong exercises very beneficial to his overall health. He had seen many different types of Qi Gong and knew they were all helpful. What was unique about the Qi Gong he did was there were preliminary warm-up techniques before the Basic Fourteen Move Qi Gong Exercise. He had taught Pei Ke the Basic Fourteen Move Qi Gong Exercise, but he had not taught him the preliminary techniques. These techniques were designed to open the acupuncture points and the meridian system so the body could benefit from the Qi Gong.

He had taught the preliminary techniques to a few students and they all agreed that the preliminary techniques substantially enhanced the Qi Gong. Because the energy was so enhanced, some felt the preliminary techniques were more important than the Qi Gong itself.

As he sat in the chair next to the table, he sipped his tea enjoying its smooth delicate flavor. He put the cup down and calmed his mind. He recited in his mind what he had been reciting for more years than he could remember.

*Suppose your head is suspended from above. String is attached to the acupuncture point Bai Hui. The string is pulling you up so you are sitting straight. Mouth is closed. Tongue touches the roof of the mouth....*

Liu continued with the process of clearing his mind and relaxing his body. He breathed in and then exhaled as he had been taught. This was in keeping with the Taoist method of breathing. Within a couple of minutes, he was ready to begin the series of Basic Moves. He enjoyed this feeling and looked forward to the expanded feeling he was going to experience in just a few minutes. There was no way he could adequately describe the relaxation he was about to experience.

The first technique was a knee exercise that strengthened the knees, ankles, and hip joints. It was a simple exercise. He shifted his body so his buttocks were towards the forward edge of the chair. With his feet flat on the floor and his knees touching, he rotated his feet in circles on the floor making sure his feet were touching the floor at all times.

One foot would go clockwise while the other foot would go counter clockwise. Looking at the feet from a seated position one would see the feet making two circles simultaneously next to each other. Then he would reverse directions. He did this flat footed and also with the heels raised about one half inch off the floor.

He knew the Yong Quan acupuncture point, which was the first point of the Kidney Meridian, would be stimulated by these circular foot movements. He attributed his strong legs, knees, and back to doing this exercise for years. He recommended the knee exercises to everyone, particularly the elderly. He had even taught it to people who had arthritic knees and ankles.  He emphasized to these arthritic patients that consistent daily practice went a long way in helping the recovery process.

The stimulation of the Yong Quan point on the Kidney Meridian would tonify the kidney energy. In males, the kidney energy was vital for a long healthy life. This was in part why he enjoyed good health when others his age were frail.

As he swirled his feet, he could feel the energy rising up the inside of his legs. He remembered when he had first learned the exercise. There was no energy rising up his legs. Instead, he felt the buildup of blood in the knees, ankles, and hips. It felt almost like they were swelling. Initially, he could only do the exercise for a short period of time because his legs would become exhausted. As time progressed, he was able to endure the initial discomfort, and now there was no discomfort—only the feeling of energy in his feet, ankles, legs, knees, and hips. It was a good feeling. It made his legs exceptionally strong and he knew that one of the secrets to being able to develop the power of Fa Jing was strong legs.

As Liu was finishing the knee exercises, Pei Ke walked into the room. At first Liu did not see him, but Pei Ke cleared his throat and Liu looked up instantly. Liu was disturbed with himself for not sensing that Pei Ke had gotten up. He was not upset that Pei Ke was watching him; rather, he was upset he was so engrossed in what he was doing that he had not sensed the energy had changed. He admonished himself for this lapse; he needed to be always on guard.

"You are up early," said Liu.

"Yes, Master. For some reason I woke up quickly and was fully alert, so I got out of bed. I see you are doing some exercise."

"Yes, since you are up, get the extra chair and sit down next to me. I want to teach you a special technique for developing internal energy. These exercises are preliminary exercises done before you do your Qi Gong exercises. They are designed to open up the important acupuncture points and to facilitate the flow of energy along the meridian system. If done correctly, you will feel the flow of the energy. It will substantially enhance the effect of the Qi Gong exercises.

"This is a unique set of exercises you probably will not see again. It is one of those things we keep dear to our heart and do not share indiscriminately with others. These exercises have been passed down to a select few over the years. One day you may want to pass them on to a select few."

"Master, where did you learn these exercises?"

"It is an accumulation of my studies with different teachers, reading of the classic books on Qi Gong, and my own insight into the how the energy in our body functions."

Pei Ke brought the chair and sat down next to Liu, feeling honored that Liu had decided to share these secrets with him. He also wondered if Liu had been getting up earlier than him to do this all this time.

Liu explained to Pei Ke what he had been doing and had Pei Ke follow along with him as he did the knee exercises for the second time.

"Master, my legs are starting to get really tired and my joints feel as if they are swelling up with blood."

"Yes, it is characteristic of this exercise technique. I know you can't do it for very long but try a little bit longer."

Pei Ke did the exercise for a few more minutes and quit. He was amazed that such an old man could do it effortlessly.

"Once you have done the knee exercises, the next step is to stimulate the acupuncture points of the knee. One of the major points is Du Bai point. It is on the Stomach Meridian and is effective in treating any type of knee problem, especially pain and swelling. It is located in the hollow below the knee cap."

Liu took Pei Ke's hand and showed him how to position the leg and knee to feel the point.

"There is another acupuncture point located just opposite Du Bai. This second point is called Xi Yan. Taken together these two points are called the 'eyes of the knee.' I want to stimulate both of these points to enhance the energy and thus enhance the strength of the knee. Watch how I stimulate these two points."

Pei Ke watched as Liu stimulated the Du Bai point with the center of his palm.

"Pay attention, Pei Ke," said Liu. "I want you to stimulate this point on your own knee exactly the way I am doing it. As I have told you, the Lao Gong acupuncture point on the center of the palm is a powerful point. Martial artists have known of this point for hundreds of years. Place your palm over the Du Bai point and move your hand exactly like I am doing. If you do it wrong, you will not get the benefit of the movement."

Pei Ke followed the directions and noticed he felt a sensation both in his palm and also in his knee. He watched as Liu stimulated the Xi Yan point, but he did it slightly differently. It appeared the Du Bai point was stimulated in one way and the Xi Yan point in another. He was about to ask Liu why it appeared there was a difference when he suddenly understood on his own. It made sense to him now. He also realized that if he stimulated the point wrong it wouldn't work.

"How do your knees feel now?" asked Liu.

"They feel strong and warm. It is a nice feeling."

"The next point I want you to know about is Yin Ling Quan. It is on the Spleen Meridian and the name means 'Yin Mound Spring.' It is one of those really important acupuncture points and has a multitude of different uses. Since it is on the Spleen Meridian, and the spleen has a tendency towards dampness and the retention of fluids in the body, this point can be used for swelling or water retention. It has a very positive effect on most pain from the middle of the body to the feet. I have used this point very often to treat lower back pain and dull achy pain residing on both sides of the lower abdominal area. Stimulating this point will help women with menstrual pain and discomfort. It will also help with the bloated feeling they have during their period. Let me show you how to locate the point and how to stimulate it."

Pei Ke watched as Liu showed him how to locate the point. Liu made a special effort to show him another point located on the opposite side of the leg. Locating one point usually made it easier to locate the other point. Liu showed Pei Ke how to stimulate the point to derive the maximum benefit.

Liu went on to show Pei Ke how to locate eight more points and how to stimulate them. It took a few minutes for Liu and Pei Ke to finish.

"How do your knees and legs feel now? Stand up and walk around."

Pei Ke walked from the chair to the door and back. He lifted up both legs and purposely put his feet on the floor.

"Master, my feet actually feel rooted to the ground. Now I am starting to grasp what you have been trying to teach me about how to root. I've heard you say many times how being rooted to the ground helps with martial arts and meditation, but I don't think I have ever felt this rooted. It's almost like my feet are now part of the ground. At the same time my feet and body feel light. It's a contradiction, I know, but I actually feel as if I can move my feet faster than before, but still stay solid and rooted."

"Good. Now sit down. There is more to learn before the villagers get up this morning. Once they are up and realize we are up, they will come for us.

"The next step in this process of preparing yourself to do Qi Gong exercises is to stimulate the Well Points. As you know, the Well Points are on the hands and feet. Here is how you stimulate them. It is very easy to do."

Pei Ke followed Liu as he stimulated the Well Points on the hands and feet. The whole process only took a minute or two.

"The next step," said Liu, "is to open up three special points. Each has a major influence on the energy of the kidneys. These three points are in close proximity to each other and can be stimulated at the same time. Pei Ke I want you to watch how I do this. You need to be careful how you do it, because it is possible to do it backwards."

Pei Ke watched and then followed exactly what Liu was doing, making sure he noted the correct way to stimulate the three points.

"Next, we stimulate the major acupuncture points on each one of the meridians. Each point has a purpose and taken together, the three hundred and sixty-one points are all important. However, there are some points that have more of an influence on the Qi of the body and therefore have a greater influence on the well-being of the body. When you stimulate these points, do it in the order I show you. This order corresponds to the circular flow of the energy in the body."

"Master, do you mean the flow of energy from one meridian to another in the twenty-four hour cycle of energy?"

"Exactly."

Liu showed Pei Ke the twelve points that were important to stimulate the flow of Qi. In essence, what Liu was showing Pei Ke was how to open the points, and thus open the energy of all the primary meridians. He showed Pei Ke how to stimulate each point, making sure he was doing it correctly.

"How do you feel now that you have stimulated all these points?"

"My body has a tingling feeling, as if the energy is flowing through my body. I still have the rooted feeling as before, but it's not as pronounced. Why is that?"

"It is still there, you just now have more energy in your body from stimulating other points. You can get up and walk around for a minute. Normally, you wouldn't walk around, but it is appropriate for you to do so as you learn. How do you feel now?"

"Actually, I feel fine. Again, I can say I feel light and when I walk I feel even lighter and more rooted to the ground. It would be nice to feel this way all the time. If these are the preliminary steps to doing the Qi Gong, I can understand why some people feel these techniques are very important in the development of internal energy. Where have these techniques come from?"

"They have been passed down from generation to generation to a select group of individuals. At one time they were only passed within a family, but now they are being taught more frequently by those who know how to do them.

"Now, the next step is to stimulate some acupuncture points on the face and scalp. This step is very old and has been done for hundreds of years. You will often see older people in the parks in Beijing and other big cities doing only these face and scalp exercises. When done properly, the exercise causes the face and scalp to feel rejuvenated. It helps to clear up your thinking and to wake you up, especially if you feel tired due to lack of sleep. Watch and follow me."

Pei Ke initially watched and then followed Liu. He watched how Liu rubbed the nose area, eyebrow area, and forehead area. Liu stopped a couple of times to correct the way Pei Ke held his hands. After a couple of tries Pei Ke could feel the stimulation in his face and scalp. He wondered how it would feel if he did it wrong and considered doing it incorrectly just to see, but he quickly dismissed the idea from his mind. He knew it would irritate Liu.

"The next step is to stimulate the energy of the ear. The classical text books say that the energy of the body goes to the ears. We know there are a few points in the ear but, unlike the body, the ear has never been fully developed as an energy pattern. Maybe someday future generations will develop and explore the ear.

"I want you to see the way I hold the ear and how I manipulate it. Start at this location and go to that location."

Liu pointed to his own ear for Pei Ke to see what direction he was suppose to go. He watched as Liu grasped his own ear and manipulated the surface of the ear. Liu placed his hand on Pei Ke's ear so he understood the amount of pressure and the manner in which the ear was to be stimulated.

"Master, it feels good. It seems to wake me up. I don't feel anything special in my body, only a generalized feeling of well being from what you just did."

"Good. The next step is to stimulate the overall flow of energy in the body. By stimulating certain major points, we have enhanced the energy along the meridian. We now want to get that enhanced energy to flow along the meridian system. As you know from your previous studies, the energy on the inside of the arm flows from the chest to the fingers and the energy on the outside of the arms flows from the fingers to the chest. This is the opposite on the legs. The energy on the inside of the legs flows from the toes to the trunk of the body, and the energy on the outside of the legs flows from the body to the toes.

"Watch how I stimulate this flow pattern."

Pei Ke watched as Liu showed him the way to move the energy along the meridian system. Pei Ke saw the pattern developing and was able to immediately follow.

"The energy in our bodies flows in a circular pattern," Liu said. "This energy influences the energy of the Conception Vessel Meridian and the Governing Vessel Meridian. These two meridians are coupled meridians just like there are coupled meridians for the Twelve Basic Meridians.

"The last acupuncture point on the Governing Vessel Meridian is Yin Jiao. It literally means 'Gum Intersection.' It is located in the mouth on the upper gum area on the outside part of the teeth where the gum intersects with the upper part of the mouth. Since all acupuncture points are located below the surface of the skin, this point is inside of the gums. In meditation, we touch the roof of the mouth with our tongue just above the gums. In doing so we are in essence touching the backside of the acupuncture point. It is easier to touch the backside of the point than it is to force our tongue to the outside of our teeth. Touching the roof of the mouth makes the connection between the Conception Vessel Meridian and the Governing vessel Meridian. We now have a complete circuit of energy.

"With the mouth closed, stimulate with your tongue the Yin Jiao point. Also stimulate all the gums and teeth, both upper and lower teeth with your tongue. Click your teeth together twenty-four times. You will notice your mouth has built up a supply of saliva. Just swallow it. This process will help your digestion."

"Master, how hard do I click my teeth?"

"It is not necessary to click your teeth very hard. It is the action of chewing that stimulates the release of saliva and that is what I want to happen. How do you feel now that you have done these preliminary exercises?

"Master, I feel wonderful and wide awake. I am ready for whatever is ahead of me for the day. It is a wonderful feeling. Can I do these exercises every day?"

"Of course. If you do them every day along with your Qi Gong and martial arts, you will stay healthy for a long time."

"Master, if I do everything you have taught me, there will be no more time to do anything else. How will I support myself, let alone support a family if I get married?"

Liu smiled as he motioned for Pei Ke to put on a coat and follow him outside. The villagers were up and by the footprints in the snow the daily activity of the village was in full swing. They were no more than a dozen feet from the front door when one of the women who had cleaned the house the day before ran up to them with her daughter in tow. She bowed in front of Liu.

"Master, is there anything you and your student need this morning? My daughter has made something for both of you. She is a very good cook. I taught her everything I know, and she learns quickly. We would be honored if you would accept this small token of our appreciation for what you have already done for this village."

The women nudged the daughter and the daughter extended a basket. It obviously had something to eat in it. The mother smiled at Pei Ke as she quickly guided the basket away from Liu and in Pei Ke's direction. Liu bowed and a somewhat speechless Pei Ke took the basket.

"Thank you, you are both very kind," said Liu. "It is not necessary for you..."

"It is our pleasure," said the woman. "If there is anything you need, please feel free to ask us; we will be happy to handle it for you. I suspect you two will be very busy today seeing some of the villagers. Why don't you both go back inside and eat your breakfast? We assumed you both are vegetarian so we prepared vegetables and rice for you."

"Actually, you have a good suggestion," said Liu.

Soon there was a long line of villagers at their door. They all talked excitedly about the doctor and his student.

Liu was impressed by the things the previous doctor had accumulated. There were enough needles, moxa, splints, and Chinese herbs to take care of patients for the day. Liu had Pei Ke make sure the needles were sterile for the day and placed in a sterile container.

Part of the time Liu did the diagnosis and part of the time he watched as Pei Ke went through the differential diagnosis process. With each patient, Liu asked Pei Ke about what he had found and helped him refine his diagnosis. Pei Ke was amazed at how much Liu could determine about what had happened to the patient just by asking a few questions. With almost every patient, there was a question Pei Ke would not have thought to ask.

During the day, he again saw Mrs. Lo and Mr. Po. They both were doing much better and were exceedingly grateful. The cases coming through the front door included what would be seen in any normal clinic, but it was overwhelming for Pei Ke. He worked continuously without a break.

One of the cases was the child Liu had seen the day before. The mother brought the child towards the end of the day.

"Master Liu, do you remember me. I was in the crowd yesterday. You looked at my baby for a second. I got the impression you could help him."

"Yes, I remember seeing you. I am glad you came today. If you had not come, I would have gone in search of you and your baby. Let me have a look at him."

The mother unwrapped the baby and handed him over to Liu. He looked at the baby's face, head, and abdomen. Liu could see the baby had lost some hair and the infant's abdomen was slightly distended.

"How long has your baby been losing hair?"

"It has been about a month now."

"How long has his abdomen been distended?"

"Same, about a month. We don't know why."

"How old is he?"

"Six months old."

"Are you nursing him?"

"I am trying to, but I do not have very much milk. I give him water to supplement my feeding him."

"Do you feed him any solid foods, or do you just nurse and supplement with water?'

"I just nurse and supplement with water."

"Is this your first child?"

"Yes."

"How old are you?"

"Twenty."

"Where do you live?"

"I live with my parents here in the village. My husband died just after my son was born. We lived southeast of here in a small village. One day the soldiers came looking for new volunteers. He resisted and was killed to make an example to the rest of the villagers. His parents had passed away and there wasn't enough room to stay with his siblings. I had no place to go so I came back to my parents."

"How long have you been here?"

"I arrived a couple of days ago. I have been traveling alone with my baby for a couple of weeks."

"You and your baby are lucky to be alive," said Liu. "Where did you stay and what did you eat while traveling?"

"Some people were nice to let me stay with them for the night, others just shunned me. I didn't often have much to eat. I made sure to drink plenty of water so I could nurse, but my milk seems to have decreased substantially. What is wrong with my baby? Can you help?"

"Pei Ke, I want you to hold the infant."

Liu put the baby into Pei Ke's hands. Pei Ke looked startled as he accepted the squirming infant. It had been a long time since he had held a baby, and he was slightly uncomfortable. He looked at Liu as he accepted the infant and Liu gave him a slight smile.

"Get used to it," said Liu. "Your time is going to come one of these days."

Liu motioned for the woman to lie on the exam table. The infant initially started to cry and Pei Ke was about to panic.

"Rock the baby in your arms for a few minutes," said Liu.

After a couple moments of rocking, the baby stopped whimpering and looked up at Pei Ke and smiled. Pei Ke smiled back and an unknown emotion swept over him. Pei Ke looked up at Liu and the woman. Both were smiling at him.

"You would make a good father," said the woman. "You should be married by now. Are you?"

"No," said Pei Ke. "Maybe someday. For now all of my time is spent learning from Master Liu."

"Have you found a woman you like?"

Pei Ke was startled by the question. He didn't know what to say. Liu looked at him and then saved him.

"Are you comfortable?" he asked the woman.

"Yes, Master," said the woman.

"How are you and the baby doing, Pei Ke?"

"I'm doing fine, Master. I guess I should say we are doing fine. The baby seems to like me. He keeps looking at my face and smiling. Maybe he thinks I know what I am doing."

"Maybe you are a natural at being a father. You should consider finding yourself a nice wife."

Pei Ke looked at Liu. Was his Master telling him something? Pei Ke was sure Liu knew how he felt about Mei Li but did he know he also thought about Hua Yee?

"I need to ask you some more questions," said Liu.

"What?" asked Pei Ke, startled. What is he going to ask me? How am I going to respond?

"Not you, Pei Ke."

"Of course," said the woman, smiling.

"Are you eating properly now that you are here with your parents?"

"Yes, my mother is taking care of me. She is making sure I have enough to eat."

Liu asked the young woman a series of questions similar to those he would ask of any woman he was examining. In addition, he asked her specific questions pertaining to her poor lactation. He went through the diagnostic process of pulse-taking and examining her tongue. He asked her many questions about the baby and then went over to Pei Ke and the baby.

"Pei Ke, there is a special way to take the pulse of an infant. Watch how I do it. The pulse of a child is usually faster than that of an adult. So you have to take this into consideration when you make your diagnosis.

Pei Ke watched as Liu took the pulses of the infant. Yes indeed there was a difference in how he examined the energy flow through the pulses.

"Pei Ke I want you to take the pulse of our patient and then the pulse of the infant as you saw me do it."

Pei Ke gently handed the infant to Liu and was turning to the woman when the infant began to cry. He looked at Liu and then again at the woman.

"He likes you," said the woman.

"Pei Ke, take the pulses."

The woman smiled as he took hold of her wrist. He took the pulses and made note of what he found. He looked at her tongue and even asked her a few questions. Next, he took the pulses of the child. He followed exactly as Liu had done.

"Pei Ke, I want you to feel the skin and muscle on the infant's legs and arms, paying close attention to the softness or hardness of the muscles, and then the same thing on the infant's abdomen."

Pei Ke did as he was instructed to do.

"Master, there is a distinct difference between the infant's arms and legs, and the abdomen. The abdomen feels as if it is bloated and the arms and legs feel flaccid."

"Yes. Did you feel the difference in the infant's pulse in comparison to what you have seen in the pulse of adults?"

"Yes."

"Master, are we going to be all right?"

"Yes, I think so."

"What's wrong?" asked the woman.

"There are two different things happening here, but both are related to the stressful situation you and your baby have undergone in the last few months. As you know, you are not producing enough milk to adequately nourish your baby. This causes one type of condition in you. The good news is you are on the right track by being with your mother who I expect knows what you need to eat and will see to it that you get the right nourishment. We are going to treat you with acupuncture and have you take some Chinese herbal formulas for a few days to get you back to where you need to be so you can nurse your baby.

"Nursing is very important for the development of your child and once we get you back to where you need to be, which shouldn't take too long, then I want you to nurse a little longer than normal. This will help your baby.

"For your baby, I suspect because your nursing has been irregular and the supply of milk has been irregular, he has developed a condition of a deficiency of spleen and stomach. The symptoms your baby exhibits with the thinning hair, protruding abdomen and belly button, thin arms and legs, dry skin, and other indications confirm the problem. The reason your baby has this problem is the inability of the spleen and stomach to do what they are intended to do because of the irregular food intake. In your case, it is the irregular nursing.

"This problem is solvable now that you are on a good diet and your milk supply should come back to normal. I am going to treat you to balance your energy and use specific points that will increase your milk output. Of course this is dependent on your new diet. For your baby, I am going to do acupuncture on him but the technique is going to be different than what I would use on an adult. Since he is so young and there is a deficiency, I am going to put the needles in, twirl them for a couple of seconds, and immediately take them out.

"I want to balance as much as possible, but I don't want to stimulate too much because of his weakened condition. I will prepare an herbal formula for him to take which should help. He doesn't need to take too much. Of course, he will only be able to take little sips. I expect both of you will return to a normal condition soon."

Pei Ke held the infant as Liu did acupuncture on the woman. He made some funny faces and could see the infant was smiling in response. He rocked the baby and twirled the baby in small circles, always watching for a response.

"Pei Ke, have you been paying attention to what I have been doing?"

"Yes, of course, Master."

"These are the acupuncture points used to increase a woman's milk supply. I will also give her some herbs that will help her to adequately nurse."

"Yes, Master. I have seen you use this combination once before."

Liu continued with the treatment process. Pei Ke watched as Liu then treated the infant.

"The first point I am going to use is Xia Wan point. This point specifically is used to balance both the stomach energy and the spleen energy simultaneously. This point is particularly effective when treating malnourished children.

"The second point is the Wei Shu point. It is one of the back Shu Points along the Urinary Bladder Meridian. As you know Wei means 'stomach' and this is one of the primary points for treating anything related to stomach disharmony.

"The third point is the Pi Shu. Pi literally means 'spleen' and this, like Wei Shu, is designed to specifically treat the energy of a specific organ. In this case, it is the spleen.

"The fourth point is Tai Bai point. This point is used to balance the energy in both the stomach and spleen."

Pei Ke watched as Liu chose other points. In each case, Liu would insert the needle and then quickly remove it. When he was done he put the infant into the woman's arms.

"How do you feel now?"

"I feel more relaxed, and it seems some of the agitation in my baby is gone. Actually, he's fallen asleep. Thank you so much. We're all so grateful. Won't you please stay and make this your home? I'm sure there are enough people here that your student will one day want to take over and make this his home."

Later that day, Liu saw the woman who had brought the morning delicacies arguing with the two other women who had helped with the cleaning. It then dawned on him there were virtually few men of Pei Ke's age in the village. The men were very young, married, or older. No wonder the mothers wanted their daughters to meet an eligible male. There were very few here and his guess was that there was no prospect for them to find one. The young girls would end up unmarried maidens.

Liu wondered what had happened to all the eligible males. A number of different possibilities went through his mind as he watched from a distance as the three women argued.

As he was debating the consequences, a prickling feeling went up his neck. He instantly turned his head to look off into the distance at the hill where he last saw what he surmised would be his adversary. As he scanned the area, he didn't see anything unusual, but there was something in the Universal Energy that caught his attention.

# CHAPTER TWENTY-SEVEN

Liu and Pei Ke stayed in the village for a few days. Early each morning, Liu would have a long line of patients waiting for him. He didn't mind taking care of them. All people were the same in his eyes. There weren't rich people and poor people. They were all part of the Universal Tao, and he needed to make sure whoever he came in contact with would be better off for that connection.

Word had spread that there was a doctor in the village and after the third day, there were more and more people he had not seen before. They came from not only the outlying areas surrounding the village, but also from other villages within a day's walk.

"Master, we have been here four days now. You have seen so many patients with a myriad of ailments. I have learned more in these four days than I have in all the time I've studied with you."

"Yes, there is no substitution for actual observation and practice. Of course, book learning is important but practical experience is where you apply what you have been taught and what you have read.

"Pei Ke, now that we have been here for a few days, what do you think of this village and the people?"

"They seem to be very nice and they pay great respect to you as a doctor."

"Would you consider living in this village?"

"I would if you would be living here. I told you I'm going to go wherever you go. If this is where you want to be, then I will stay as well."

"Someday you are going to be a doctor and practice on your own. Would you consider this village?"

"I don't want to completely eliminate the possibility, but right now I don't think this place gives me the things I want. It is too small and too isolated from other places."

"You have made an impression with the villagers. If you ever come this way again, be sure and visit with the them. They will remember both of us, and your opinion about staying here may change over time.

"We are going to be leaving here in the morning and continue on to Beijing. We have stayed long enough and you have benefited tremendously from the opportunity to treat these people."

"Master, do you feel these people will be safe once we leave?"

"Hopefully, they will not have any more problems. Maybe we can check on them if we return this way. For now we must be on our way."

That night Liu and Pei Ke visited with the elders and many of the patients they had treated. Liu explained that they must be on their way. He thanked them for their hospitality and promised that if they ever came back, they would make a point of staying with them again. The villagers used every possible tactic to get them to stay, but Liu was adamant about continuing on their journey.

During the night, the temperature dropped again and two to three inches of fresh snow fell. In the morning, Liu and Pei Ke were up early. After taking tea and doing their Qi Gong exercises, they were on their way. As they walked away from the village, Liu saw footsteps in the snow. They came from outside the village, away from where Liu and Pei Ke were staying. Liu turned to look back and could see their own footsteps in the snow. They merged with those that came from beyond, which continued on in the direction of Beijing.

Liu was uneasy with this coincidence. He sensed he and Pei Ke would soon meet up with those he had seen on the hill days before.

Chen Chang watched that early morning as Liu and Pei Ke headed out from the village. He wanted to attack as soon as possible, but he wanted to make sure Liu and Pei Ke were away from the village. He didn't want the villagers to interfere. Would it be better to attack while Liu was in the countryside or to wait for Liu to get to Beijing, where he could entice others to help him? He was deep in thought as he lost sight of Liu and Pei Ke.

# CHAPTER TWENTY-EIGHT

The following morning they found themselves traveling through a dense pine forest. Liu looked at the trees and recognized the specific variety. He had seen it many times before in the mountains surrounding his boyhood home. He could smell the richness of the scent. He remembered his father taking him into the woods on many different occasions and teaching him the ways of the forest.

He'd learned about the animals and the clues they left behind. He could tell the type of animal by the foot prints, fur, and droppings. He could tell the approximate weight and age of the animal by the shape and depth of the foot print. He could tell if the animal was wounded or hurt by the spacing of the trail it left. He smiled inwardly as he reminisced about his childhood. He was abruptly brought out of his reverie by Pei Ke's question.

"Master, we have talked about the Tao and Taoism. It seems Taoism is both a philosophy and a religion. This seems different from Confucianism, which is a moral structure we follow and Buddhism, which is a religion founded by Buddha. How do you visualize the philosophy of Tao?"

"There are many different religions in this universe. When I was visiting in Beijing and later in Shanghai, I was introduced to philosophies and religions I had never heard of before. There is a common thread in most philosophies and religions.

"Basically, there is the concept of being good, doing good deeds, and treating everyone with respect. The various religions pursue this concept differently because different religious leaders have made an impact on their followers.

"Almost always, these religions thrive because of the existence of an authority figure, who guides the group toward an accepted goal.

"Some individuals find that Taoist philosophy provides what they need in order to have peace within themselves. Taoism adheres to the principles of the Tao, but it is given structure by Taoist priests performing ceremonial activities. The ceremonial activities bind the practitioners together and give them a sense of belonging, which is a common requirement of society.

"I lived at the temple not because it provided a common singular religious experience, but because the temple specifically did not adhere to a dogma constraining me to a specific belief, and that opened me up to explore the vast teachings of many different religions and philosophies."

"Master, would you recommend someone join a Taoist or a Buddhist temple?"

"Each person is different and should follow whatever they think is best for them. What seems to be a universal truth is that most people feel better in the company of like-minded individuals, and feel better if they have a common social surrounding and goals. Most religious organizations have projects or goals to bring people together. Without the goals or dogma, participants have a tendency to stray away from the established beliefs."

"Master, you speak so often of the Universal Tao and the energy associated with the Tao. Religious Taoism must have these same concepts plus more."

"Religious Taoism is for those who want to have cohesiveness to their worship. The Taoist priests, through their incantations and ceremonial activities, satisfy the requirements of the practitioners. The individual practice of Taoism does not have any of the ceremonial activities of religious Taoism."

"Is one better than the other?" asked Pei Ke.

"It depends on what you want and how you were brought up as a child. My choice, not to be part of the religious aspect of Taoism, is purely my own, but there are others who have gained much from the religious aspect of it, and I am very happy for them, for it has given them some direction in life.

"At the same time, even though these religious organizations give direction to the person's life, they need to be careful that the organization does not take on concepts detrimental to the individual or others who may not believe the same. We see this quite often when there are shifts in the ruling powers of China, especially in the countryside where a ruler has decided to change from one belief to another and forces others to follow. It can become quite disconcerting for the populace when this happens."

"Master, are there more people who follow Buddhism or Taoism?"

"Taoism is native to China. Buddhism is native to India, but was brought here by Buddha. Buddhism, as I mentioned a few minutes ago, gives the practitioner an opportunity to be part of a cohesive group of like-minded people. True Taoism is a totally individual form of philosophy that downplays the interaction within a group. There are far more Buddhists than there are Taoists. Neither one is right or wrong. I believe in both and hold both in high regard. However, if you look at the internal martial arts, they can be classified as Taoist because they rely more on the internal aspect of the human and the energy the human can generate. This concept of energy is not as prevalent in Buddhism."

Pei Ke pondered this. He wondered if he should be a Buddhist or a Taoist. His parents were both Buddhist. He had gone to the Buddhist temple with his mother and had performed some of the rituals. He'd thought it was boring, but it had been important for his mother.

Liu continued to think about his boyhood activities with his parents. He acknowledged what his parents had done in bringing up their children. He was saddened he would never have children of his own to pass on the teachings his parents had given him. He looked at Pei Ke. The boy was truly innocent in his personal way of life. Liu smiled to himself as he picked up the pace. Pei Ke sped up to follow.

# CHAPTER TWENTY-NINE

They walked for a couple of days. They often found shelter with one or more of the local residents. The weather was now colder with snow flurries in the air even on the lower elevations of their travels. Pei Ke was sure the residents took pity on them in the cold winter environment and didn't want them to sleep on the ground.

Each day, Liu drilled Pei Ke on the fine art of Pa Kua Chang. Occasionally, he would show him Chin Na techniques and some grappling. Almost every day, Pei Ke did strength building exercises as they walked. Pei Ke had long ago dismissed the ridiculousness of these moves. He knew how stupid it looked for him to have his arms stretched out at an angle in the customary Pa Kua Chang move, but he knew he was developing a tremendous amount of strength in his shoulders and upper body.

Liu asked Pei Ke to stretch out his arms. Liu touched Pei Ke's shoulder and felt an indentation in the shoulder muscle where the shoulder was attached to the body.

"Pei Ke, with your right arm stretched out I want you to feel this location on your shoulder."

Pei Ke did as Liu instructed. He had done this before.

"Do you remember when I had you first feel the indentation on my shoulder and the lack of an indentation on your shoulder?"

"Yes, Master, I remember."

"Those of us who practice Pa Kua Chang almost universally have this indentation in the shoulder muscle. This is good. It indicates your upper body and shoulders are becoming strong."

Pei Ke could feel the indentation was even more pronounced than it had been before. He also knew his shoulders were becoming stronger because he could do many of the martial arts postures without experiencing any discomfort. He remembered when he had initially started learning these movements, they were almost impossible for him to do.

"Pei Ke, the benefit of the strength you are developing from doing Pa Kua Chang will carry over to Hsing-Yi Chuan. Until now I have only shown you a little Hsing-Yi Chuan."

"Master, you have mentioned there are Five Elements, you have shown me their movements, but you have not shown them in detail. When we were visiting with Wei Ken De, Mei Li showed me the Hsing-Yi Chuan her father was teaching her. It is not as beautiful as Pa Kua Chang, but it looks very explosive and powerful. When will you teach me more?"

"I showed you a stepping pattern some time ago. In fact I have had you practice this pattern many times since we initially began our travels. I know you don't realize it but I have also taught you fist patterns that you have been practicing for quite some time. When you combine one of the step patterns and one of the fist patterns it becomes Pi Chuan in Hsing-Yi Chuan, which roughly means 'splitting.' You will understand the movement when you understand the application. The total movement is done like this."

Liu brought his hands to his hips and then both hands rose simultaneously from the center of his body. The hands moved together, but the right hand was ahead of the left and the left hand was near to the inside of the right elbow. Once the right fist was fully extended upward at an angle, it retreated back and there was a follow through with the left hand. As the hands were moving so were the feet. The hands and feet were coordinated with each other.

"Pei Ke, the Pi Chuan movement is both a defensive and an offensive move in one single movement. Put your right fist in front of my face."

Pei Ke did as he was instructed. As his fist went towards Liu's face, Liu executed the Pi Chuan movement. He blocked Pei Ke's fist and the follow through with his other hand landed on Pei Ke's collar bone with a tremendous jolt. It stunned Pei Ke, and he felt as if something had penetrated his upper body.

"Are you hurt?" asked Liu.

"No, Master, but I didn't quite expect it. Does it always feel so powerful?"

"I did it quite softly so as not to hurt you. If I had done it as I normally would, it would have split your collar bone. The move is very simple, but the effect is devastating to the opponent. Of course, it has to be done correctly for it to be effective. As always, there is a right way and a wrong way to do the movement.

"Here are some basic things you need to remember. The weight is primarily on the back leg, with a seventy thirty relationship between the back and front legs. The mind drives the movements. The movements are linear. However, as the arms move forward in a linear direction there is a simultaneous rotational direction to both arms. You can feel this rotational direction by putting your hands on my upper back."

Liu positioned Pei Ke's hands on his upper back and went through the Pi Chuan movement.

"Master, I can feel the area you are referring to. It moves as you move."

"Yes, in Chinese medicine, this acupuncture point you are feeling is a meeting point for energy in the body. If you look at the ancient acupuncture charts, you will see where this energy meeting point actually exists. I believe this meeting point is important for both martial artists and acupuncturists. You need to remember this point."

"Master, this is the same point you showed me when I was first learning Qi Gong Basic Exercises."

"Yes, you are correct. I want you to watch how I do the Pi Chuan movement. I want you to pay close attention to the coordination between the various parts of my body."

Pei Ke watched as Liu went through numerous repetitions of Pi Chuan first to the left and then to the right. He watched as Liu coordinated the back foot with the follow through of hand. There was always a foot and a hand moving in unison, with them both starting at the same time and ending at the same time. It was truly simple, but the overall coordination of Liu's body was amazing. It was fascinating how simple the movement was and yet how destructive it could be.

His mind flashed back to Mei Li. He remembered watching her do this same movement. It looked the same, but he could see that Liu had more power. Mei Li was good because of the constant drilling of her father who had learned Hsing-Yi Chuan from Liu, but she was in no way close to what Liu was showing him now. He wondered just how good Wei Ken De was. He really enjoyed doing Pa Kua Chang and had learned many of the palm changes and forms, but he also wanted to learn Hsing-Yi Chuan, mainly for the explosive power it generated.

"Master, how do you generate the power? It seems effortless, but I can see you are really rooted to the ground."

"The power of Hsing-Yi Chuan is developed through the legs. Think of the legs as springs that are compressed and then suddenly released. There is a powerful upward force as the spring expands. This is one way for you to think of the power of Hsing-Yi Chuan. We need strong legs when we do Chinese internal martial arts."

"Does it have anything to do with my weight?"

"You have seen Tai Chi Chuan, Pa Kua Chang, and Hsing-Yi Chuan. Anyone of any height or weight can do any of the three; however, each one has a characteristic a little more conducive to certain body styles. As an example, when you see the fast coiling movements of Pa Kua Chang, would you expect a heavy person or a thin person to be faster in the movements?"

"Master, I would expect someone short and thin would be able to do the turning and coiling much better than someone that was heavier."

"Correct, but it doesn't mean someone who is heavy cannot be good at Pa Kua Chang. Some of the best Pa Kua Chang practitioners are heavy, and they can be very formidable opponents.

"From what you have seen with Hsing-Yi Chuan, would you expect the best practitioners to be tall and thin?"

"Master, based on what I have seen you do, I would expect the best practitioners to be heavier than the Pa Kua Chang practitioners."

"Yes, you are correct, but again it doesn't mean there are not any really good, thin Hsing-Yi Chuan practitioners. Using the explosive power of Hsing-Yi Chuan coupled with the mass of the body produces a very formidable opponent. Now, what would you expect with a Tai Chi Chuan practitioner?"

"Master, I have not seen enough Tai Chi Chuan to answer the question."

"In my opinion weight doesn't matter, but height does. Those who are tall don't have a low center of gravity and can be upended more easily than those with a low center of gravity."

"Are you suggesting that for me to do Hsing-Yi Chuan well I need to put on some weight?"

"No, you want to be just the way you are. You will find over time you will have an affinity for one or more of these three arts. It doesn't mean you should ignore the others. What is more important is for you to be able to switch from one to the other in a split second. That way you can use the type of martial art to fit the situation. In addition, it will slightly confuse your opponent who will have to adjust to the ever changing style."

For the rest of their travels Pei Ke always took some time during the day to practice the Pi Chuan movements.

# CHAPTER THIRTY

Eyes followed Liu and Pei Ke as they walked through the countryside. Liu had been more aware of them the last couple of days. At first they were distant, but now he sensed their proximity. He couldn't decide if what he was feeling was reality or his growing concern that something sinister was about to take place.

His thoughts turned to the events since he and Pei Ke had left on their journey to his ancestral home. The travels north, the meeting with Hou and We Ken De, and the emotional meeting with Hua Yee, his niece, flooded through his mind one after another.

As they walked, he turned to briefly look at Pei Ke. Pei Ke was young and had his whole life ahead of him. Pei Ke had learned a lot in a short period of time. His knowledge of Chinese medicine was improving every day. In a couple of years, he would be able to have his own patients. But his martial arts ability was not keeping up with his true abilities. Liu couldn't decide if it was too much for Pei Ke to learn or Pei Ke had really more of an affinity for medicine. He had questioned Pei Ke numerous times trying to determine where his student's interest was headed, but each time he asked, Pei Ke had indicated he wanted to learn everything.

Liu realized that over the course of his own lifetime, he had had many different teachers. Each of these teachers had been the best he could find at the time. Pei Ke so far had only had one teacher, so to some extent the teaching has been biased.

Maybe it was time to really focus on just one thing. Pei Ke was getting a smattering of many different things to keep up his interest, but maybe it was not what was needed now. Maybe he should send Pei Ke to Wei Ken De and let him study awhile with his inner door student. Wei Ken De was a very good martial artist. In fact Wei Ken De's Hsing-Yi Chuan was unbelievably good. He felt one day Wei Ken De would probably be better than he was.

Liu again thought about this journey he was making to Beijing. He wanted to meet with some of his former friends and acquaintances. He had not been there for years and wondered once more if he would even be able to find them. If he couldn't find any of them, at least it would be an opportunity for Pei Ke to see places he had never seen before.

Once more he sensed they were being watched from afar. The energy was not positive, but full of hate and anger. As he was focusing on the energy, he realized there was more than one source to the energy. The energy of the eyes was following him, and the energy of the person with the hate and anger was following him also. They were on opposite sides of the road. Neither one of them was moving; rather, they were just waiting for him and Pei Ke to arrive at a particular location.

Liu stopped abruptly and motioned for Pei Ke to follow him off the road into the bamboo forest. The forest was dense as they moved farther and farther away from the road. He had chosen the side of the hateful energy. The eyes were an unknown, but he was certain the hateful energy was from Chen Chang and his band of followers. He wondered what promises had been made to these men to entice them to follow him this far. Most likely Chen Chang had told them there was a treasure, and that they would all share in it once they had killed Liu.

Of course, once Liu was dead, there couldn't be any witnesses, so it was obvious Pei Ke would have to go. Liu was amazed at the lack of moral structure within some members of society. They had no qualms about hurting others.

Pei Ke looked quizzically at Liu. Liu gestured for him to be quiet and just follow. They went deeper into the forest. Liu wanted to get around to the other side of those who were waiting for him. He didn't want to have an altercation on the road today. He knew it was coming, but today was not the day he wanted it to happen. He didn't want to have to meet up with two sets of evil energy at the same time.

The trek through the forest wasn't easy for either of them. The terrain changed from being level and smooth to rocky and slanting. They held on to the bamboo as they climbed. Liu had the leg strength, but not the endurance. Pei Ke because of his age had the endurance, but not quite the leg strength.

After twenty minutes of climbing, they reached a grassy plateau overlooking the road. Turning left they walked quickly through the knee high grass.

"Pei Ke, there are men on both sides of the road who want to do us some harm. This is why I climbed to this higher elevation. I wanted to avoid any possible altercation."

From previous experience, Pei Ke knew Liu had this uncanny ability to sense not only energy, but the quality of the energy. If it was good energy, Liu would react one way. If the energy was evil, Liu would react another way. Pei Ke knew it was better not to ask. If Liu wanted to share anything with him, he would.

They walked along the plateau for about an hour when Liu stopped and looked in the direction of the road. He looked back in the direction they had just come and then in the direction of where they were headed.

Liu was not able to sense any of the evil energy he had sensed an hour earlier. He didn't even sense the energy of whatever had been following him for so long. He motioned for Pei Ke to follow him as he descended from the plateau towards the road again. Going downhill was much easier than going uphill and they descended quite quickly to the road and continued their journey to Beijing.

# CHAPTER THIRTY-ONE

t was early morning, just before sunrise, as Liu jumped up from a deep sleep. He didn't often just jump up from such a deep sleep, but what he felt in his body and especially in the deeper reaches of his body was more than a bad dream. It was an overpowering and foreboding feeling that something sinister was going to happen, and happen soon.

He quickly looked around the small, sparsely furnished room where he and Pei Ke were staying for the night. The room was actually a small shed with furniture. There was nothing unusual about the surroundings. There was a table and a couple of chairs. A stove was in one corner, its heat almost given out for the night. All was just as it had been when they'd gone to sleep. The door was still closed and the windows seemed to be locked.

Liu looked over to see Pei Ke sound asleep on the floor. Even though everything looked normal, there was something uncanny about the room. It took a few moments before he realized that shadows were moving slowly across the room, even though there was no one else in the room but the two of them. He realized the shadows were caused by someone walking outside who was changing the intensity of the light that shown through the cracks in the window sill.

He couldn't tell if there were one or more individuals outside. He listened intently, but didn't hear anything unusual. Slowly he moved over to where Pei Ke was sleeping on the floor and nudged him gently. Pei Ke turned and Liu gestured with his finger for him to be quiet and get up.

They had sought shelter earlier than usual, about midday, as the weather was turning colder and snowflakes were starting to fall. Liu had not wanted them to be caught out in the open without some kind of protection from what he had thought was going to be a cold, brutal evening.

The village they were passing through was typical of villages in the area. After many inquiries, they found a family willing to exchange a little food and a place to sleep for someone to chop wood. Pei Ke was so used to chopping firewood, he developed a routine to expedite the process. He'd noticed that what had once been a physical strain was now rather easy. Chopping was nothing more than developing a little strength and knowing the technique of using your waist and the coordination of various parts of the body.

As usual, Pei Ke had chopped and Liu had done his best to help anyone with their health care issues. At first, the husband and wife were hesitant to discuss anything with Liu, but as the evening progressed, they had indicated their problems and Liu was able to help them. They had been deeply grateful for the help.

Liu's immediate attention was the shadows outside the window. He didn't want to have a fight if he could avoid it. He motioned for Pei Ke to follow him. They both looked through the crack in the sill and were relieved to see the shadows were nothing more than Mr. Pan the farmer going to and from the barn where the livestock were kept in cold weather.

"Master, I had a strange dream last night. I dreamt you and I were traveling. We were on the outskirts of Beijing when we were confronted by a group of men. The men attacked us from all sides and a fight started. What does the dream mean?"

Liu thought for a minute and wondered if his feeling about something sinister happening in the immediate future had anything to do with Pei Ke's dream.

"Pei Ke, were we able to defeat the attackers?" asked Liu

"There were five of them as I remember. Two attacked me and three attacked you. The two who attacked me must not have known martial arts for they seemed very slow and unbalanced in their movements. One grabbed me on the wrist and the other tried to grab me on the shoulders. I remember turning into the attack as much as possible and using a Chin Na technique to get out of the wrist grab. I turned to make a ball with my right hand above my left, centered at the midpoint of my waist. In my dream, I even remembered to tuck in my elbows and move my shoulders to the correct position. At that moment you woke me up."

"In your dream, what was I doing?"

"I don't know. I was too busy defending myself."

Liu looked at Pei Ke and was pleased. Pei Ke might just be a martial artist after all. There was a knock on the door. Pei Ke started to move towards the door when Liu touched his shoulder.

"I will get it," said Liu.

Liu opened the door a couple of inches, but kept his left foot braced against the bottom of the door in case he needed to quickly close the door.

"Master Liu, do you want to join us for breakfast?" asked Mr. Pan.

"Yes, we would like that very much. Just give us a couple of minutes and we will be there."

A few minutes later, Liu and Pei Ke walked out the door and turned towards Mr. Pan's house. Liu could see the tracks in the snow where Pan had been walking back and forth. He glanced over the area leading from the road to the farm. In the distance, he could see additional prints in the snow. He couldn't tell how many pairs of prints exactly, but from the way the snow was disturbed, there were more than just a couple of people out walking during the snow storm.

———

Breakfast was very enjoyable for Liu and Pei Ke. A hot meal with vegetable-stuffed buns and hot tea was a welcome change from some of the things they had eaten in previous mornings.

"Master, I have a question," said Mr. Pan.

"Yes?"

"Have you treated couples who cannot have children?"

"Yes, I have treated this problem quite successfully."

"Can you elaborate on your experience in solving this problem?"

"In Traditional Chinese Medicine, there are many different reasons why couples cannot have children. From my experience, the problem is not always with the woman; it can also be a problem with the husband. Unfortunately, for generations the woman has been the sole blame for not being able to produce offspring.

"It is very difficult for the husband to sometimes consider that he is the problem, so I approach it from the point of view of the woman and ask the husband to assist in the process. In this way, the husband does not feel he is to blame for what is considered only a female problem.

"I ask both the husband and wife to see me. I do this with them together and with them individually. I explain to the couple that I am going to make her jade palace more fruitful and his essence like the essence of the gods. Of course each one is happy knowing there is a greater chance for conception. Each one of them is going to have to take Chinese herbs. In addition, the woman is going to have to have a series of acupuncture treatments spread out over a few weeks."

"I assume you do a differential diagnosis with both the husband and wife, like you did last night with us?"

"Of course," said Liu.

"What is the typical problem couples have when the woman cannot conceive?"

"For the woman, it is generally one of eight to ten possible problems. There are not as many possible problems for the husband. In general with the males, I try to increase the quantity of their essence and increase their libido. With the increased libido, the husband feels that it is not his problem but he is helping with the process."

"Master, what has been your success rate in helping couples conceive?"

"Success varies from couple to couple, but as long as there is no severe injury to either the husband or the wife, I have a very high success rate in solving these kinds of problems. Of course, they both need to follow my instructions very closely and not get discouraged. Diet and stress are two of the main factors we need to deal with in these situations."

"Master, can you tell me from a Traditional Chinese Medicine point of view what the main causes are for infertility in a woman? I know you mentioned there were possibly eight to ten different reasons."

Liu went on to briefly describe the many possible reasons for the infertility problem. Pei Ke listened intently. He sensed Liu was giving him the information rather than Mr. Pan. An hour later, Liu thanked them for their hospitality. Liu suggested that if the couple knows of anyone who has such a problem, Traditional Chinese Medicine has helped most couples in their quest to have children. He went on to tell them that in many instances, the process is quick, with very little cost.

As Liu and Pei Ke walked away from Mr. Pan's house Liu saw even more foot prints in the snow. They turned to the right and continued on towards Beijing.

# CHAPTER THIRTY-TWO

They had walked through the snow for only a few minutes when Pei Ke turned to Liu.

"Master, may I ask you a question?"

Liu looked at the foot prints in the snow and then looked to the left and right. He did not see or sense anything out of the ordinary. Maybe his feeling in the early morning was wrong.

"What is the question about?"

"I know we've covered this topic before when we treated Mr. Po. It concerns a problem my mother had. She often complained of insomnia. Would you elaborate more on this? I am curious about the causes and treatment of this problem."

"What do you think is the problem?"

Without hesitancy Pei Ke replied.

"It is like all problems we have as humans; it is an imbalance of energy in the body. When we correct the imbalance, then the body will return to a normal condition."

"Where would you expect the imbalance to lie?"

"We would not know until we examined the patient. Once we examined the patient, we can come up with our differential diagnosis."

"Would you expect the insomnia to be a lung problem?"

"No, I would expect this to be probably a heart problem, since the heart has to do with many activities of the mind."

"Very good. To answer your question, insomnia can be due to a number of problems, but typically it is related to a dysfunction of the energy associated with heart, liver, spleen, or kidney. As I mentioned before it does not mean there is anything wrong with the specific organ. It is the energy on the meridian that causes the problem.

"Typically, the patient will indicate difficulty falling asleep, or waking up soon after falling asleep, or waking up numerous times during the night, or an inability to fall asleep at all. Because of the nature of the problem, patients might complain of light-headedness, headache, heart palpitations, the inability to remember things, and various mental or emotional problems."

"Master, what actually causes the problem? Is it a physical problem or mental problem?"

"Pei Ke, have you ever laid in bed and struggled to go to sleep because you were anxious about something?"

"Of course, doesn't that happen to everyone at one time or another?"

"Yes, but it can become chronic; and it is one reason for the insomnia.

"Insomnia can be due to situations where we are overly anxious or we have too many mental activities or feel we are working too many hours. Our minds become disturbed and do not get a chance to rest.

"Insomnia can also be caused by too many bedroom activities, extended periods of chronic sickness or illness, or even a genetic factor passed on from one's ancestors.

"In addition, the food we eat can have a major impact on the insomnia. This is especially true when there is irregular food intake. We see this when people work extended and irregular hours and don't eat their meals at scheduled times during the day. This is what happened to Mr. Po.

"Emotional factors such as depression can have an adverse effect on the liver energy causing the Qi to rise upwards, which also can cause the symptoms of insomnia."

"Master, how do we differentiate between these various causative factors?"

"Pei Ke, we know, or I should say our ancestors have known, specific signs and symptoms for us to look for to be able to identify the problem and determine how to treat it.

"As an example, if the patient has difficulty each night falling asleep, we might suspect a heart and spleen Qi involvement leading to deficiency. We can further clarify this if the patient tells us his sleep is disturbed by dreams. We would expect to hear from the patient about his bad memory and lack of motivation. I would expect his tongue to be pale and his pulse to be deficient.

"As you can see, and as you noted, the heart is involved in this insomnia. If instead of the spleen being involved the kidney is involved, then we would have a different set of signs and symptoms."

"Master, what would those symptoms be?"

"If the heart and kidney are involved in the insomnia, we would expect to see complaints related to the ear and mouth, such as tinnitus and dry mouth. There may even be some dizziness. Since the heart is involved, we might hear the patient complain of a burning sensation in the hands and feet. I would expect the tongue to be red. The patient's pulse would probably be fast and thin. Since the kidney is involved, there might even be some low-grade back pain."

"Master, I remember you telling me before about the kidney and the kidney energy. Reflecting back on what you previously mentioned, it seems that many times when there is a kidney involvement, there is a low back pain issue. Is that true?"

"You cannot say that for every time there is a kidney involvement there is low back pain. However, you are correct in saying there is a strong correlation between back pain and kidney involvement. You have made a good observation.

"Pei Ke, there are a couple more factors for me to mention to you concerning insomnia. Sometimes insomnia is due to the upward migration of Liver Fire. The energy causes the patient to have headaches, and restless, dream-disturbed sleeping patterns. Since the liver is involved in the insomnia, the patient might complain of a taste in the mouth.

"Pei Ke, if the liver is involved and the patient complains of a distinct taste in the mouth, what would you expect the patient to tell you? Would it be a sweet taste or a hot taste?"

"Master, since liver deals with sour or bitter things, it would be neither of those. The patient would probably complain of a sour or bitter taste."

"Very good."

Pei Ke smiled inwardly. He was happy he could answer the question without any hesitancy. It was a good feeling.

"Pei Ke, in addition to what I have also mentioned, insomnia can be caused by a dysfunction of the stomach. When this happens, the patient often feels pain in the abdominal area. Complaints of belching are common. We would expect the tongue to have a sticky coating on it. There would be a rolling pulse instead of a thready pulse. The patient might even indicate his bowel movements contain some undigested food.

"Pei Ke these are the basic indications of insomnia. There are more, but you will find that the majority of cases fall into these categories."

"Master, once we know the signs and symptoms; how do we treat the problem?"

"In some instances, it can require nothing more than a life style change. This is especially true if the patient is overworked or is studying too many hours. Changing an erratic eating schedule or even limiting the intake of food to early evening hours may be of some help.

"Did your mother have an erratic lifestyle?"

"No," said Pei Ke. "She probably falls into the category of a liver imbalance. She was frequently depressed. I think it had to do with the family always wondering how we would make it from one year to another. Both my parents worked hard, but we really did not have very much, and I know it bothered my mother quite a bit.

"Pei Ke, to treat this problem of insomnia we can use either acupuncture or Chinese herbal formulations or both. If we use acupuncture, can you think of how we would do it?"

"You mean how to choose the points?"

"Yes."

"Master, once we decided on the cause I suppose we would use points along the specific meridians. The heart, kidney, liver, and spleen would be involved. I would choose points dealing with those meridians."

"Good. If there was a heart involvement, which point on which meridian would you choose?"

Pei Ke thought for a few moments. His mind flashed back to the example Liu had given him some time ago concerning a tree falling in a forest blocking the water. Not only could the water not go downstream, but it was backed up causing congestion upstream.

"Master, it is possible for us to use points on the specific meridians involved. We could also use points on other meridians. I suspect the Bladder Meridian might have some points useful to treating insomnia."

"Good. Pay attention and I will tell you the points to use for each one of these situations. The information I am going to give you is in addition to what you might read or hear from other sources."

As they walked along the road, Liu explained to Pei Ke the various points and the rational for using each of them. He compared the traditional choice of points and his choice of points.

"Master, how do I determine which set of points to use?"

"Each doctor makes his decision on his accumulated knowledge and clinical experience. Quite often the decision comes down to a differentiation between one symptom and another. You may someday come across a situation where you can treat the patient using your own experience."

"Master, since you have been practicing Traditional Chinese Medicine for so many years you probably have many methods you use that other doctors do not. Is that correct?"

"Yes, I have many techniques that are not documented in the classical writings. This is true of other doctors who have been practicing as long as I have. When you find other knowledgeable doctors, they may or may not want to share their information. I have always been open with what I have learned, but I am a rarity."

"Master, why is it that some doctors share their experience and other doctors do not?"

"Each doctor has his own reasons for sharing or not sharing. I share with you and others because I want to shorten your learning process and further the body of knowledge. I suspect those doctors who do not share their learned experience do so out of a desire to have a competitive edge over other doctors."

Pei Ke thought about what Liu had said as the two of them walked along the road. They walked on, but after a hundred yards or so, Liu stopped and looked off into the distance. He knew something was not right, as the Universal Energy had changed from peacefulness to anguish. He didn't know why it had changed but he had experienced it so many times in his life, he knew there was something ahead that would change the direction of his travels.

He looked at Pei Ke and decided not to mention anything to him. He knew that one day, Pei Ke would also have the insight to sense changes in the Universal Energy. Pei Ke was not there yet, but he was getting close.

# CHAPTER THIRTY-THREE

Liu estimated they were no more than two days travel from Beijing. As they neared the city, the countryside took on less of a rustic appearance. There were more farms, and they looked more productive than some of the farms they saw in the remote areas. Liu suspected that most of the farm products produced in the surrounding area went to the city to support the never-ending appetite of the populace.

"Master."

"Yes."

"We've been walking for quite a few miles today. You've been very quiet."

"I have been deep in thought, thinking mainly of my family and Hua Yee. She is very nice and so young to be without her family. She is almost of the age where she can get married. I was thinking of the various families in the area, and if there were any suitable young men who would be appropriate for her."

Liu turned his head slightly to look at Pei Ke as they walked along the road. Pei Ke returned the look and didn't know what to say.

Pei Ke didn't know if Liu wanted a response or, if he did, what the response was supposed to be. His thoughts quickly went to Hua Yee and Mei Li. Mei Li was older than Hua Yee. Mei Li practiced martial arts. Hua Yee didn't practice martial arts, but she was the niece of Liu. Marrying Hua Yee would automatically solidify his position within the Liu family and immediately give him money and status.

However, Liu would not be alive forever and marrying Mei Li would insure that if anything happened to Liu, Pei Ke would be able to continue his studies with her father, Wei Ken De.

Both Hua Yee and Mei Li had charming attributes. They both smiled a lot, and they both could carry on a conversation. Mei Li was more self-assured and outgoing because she had been brought up by her father to be self sufficient. The death of her mother had thrust a lot of responsibilities her way. To her credit she stepped forward and assumed those responsibilities admirably.

Hua Yee was more reserved, which was to be expected coming from such a well-known family that adhered to the old customs and traditions. There was something to be said for a wife who would carry on the traditions and insure that the family structure would remain intact. Marrying Hua Yee would give him access to the Liu estate.

It was an interesting dilemma for him at this junction in his life. He had been told by those who could look into the future that his life would be interesting and that he would need to make many hard decisions. He realized that he had made more serious decisions in the last few months than he had made in his whole life up to this time.

"Pei Ke, have you given any thought as to when you would like to get married?"

"It has crossed my mind on occasion."

Pei Ke made sure he spoke carefully. He knew that Liu was probing with his questions. He didn't want to say the wrong thing.

"Master, what do you think I should do?"

"It all depends on you. What do you want to accomplish in life?"

"Right now all I want to do is to learn martial arts and medicine from you. That's why I followed you when you left the temple."

Liu contemplated Pei Ke's answer and thought of his own travels through life—what he had given up and what he had gained from his life of austerity. No matter how he evaluated it and no matter how many times he had thought through his life's journey, he knew he had made the right decision. He knew, though that his decision was his alone, and he could not expect someone else to follow in his exact footsteps. He thought of the process he had gone through in each step of his life. He had had to make many decisions, and each seemed to have been the right decision. Almost all the decisions he had made were life changing. He remembered when he'd decided to explore the internal martial arts of Tai Chi Chuan, Pa Kua Chang, and Hsing-Yi Chuan. He'd already known his family's martial arts and that would have been enough for him to handle many altercations. When the situation presented itself, however, he'd immediately grasped the opportunity. He thought of where he would be today and what he would be doing if he had only continued to study those arts he already knew.

There had also been the opportunity to advance his studies in Chinese medicine. If he hadn't made his initial trip to Beijing, he would not have had the opportunity to study from some of the best in the world. So his thoughts turned to their pending arrival in Beijing. He had not been back for quite some time and he was anxious to meet up with whoever he could find. There had been many upheavals in the land and of course the politics of the emperor change like the changing wind.

He guessed the city would be different, but he had been there for long enough the first time that he was confident once he was inside the walls of the city he would be able to find his way around.

His thoughts turned back to Pei Ke. Would Pei Ke make the right decisions in life or would he be led astray by extraneous factors? He thought Pei Ke had made the right decision by not causing the secret of the Liu fortune to be opened for all to see. Once the information about the passing of the Liu fortune had been made known, then the vultures would descend upon those who had inherited the fortune. He was sure the situation with the title of the land was correct but Chen Chang was still at large and he was positive once Chen knew of the extent of the fortune, he would try to assert his claim, even though his father was dead. The greed would be too much for him and another attack would be forthcoming. At least for now the secret was safe, and he only needed to deal with someone who was seeking revenge.

"Pei Ke, do you still carry the amulet I gave you?"

"Of course, Master. Do you want it back?"

"Yes, give it back to me."

Without hesitation Pei Ke unbuttoned his tunic and pulled out the broken amulet. Looking at it, no one would ever guess it controlled a fortune.

He gave it to Liu without any hesitation. He was surprised that it didn't bother him to give it up, knowing that only a few days earlier he could have given the amulet to the Abbot at the temple and the Abbot would have given him his portion of the treasure.

He did not know what the treasure was, but from all the mystery and caution, he thought it must be immense. He guessed the amulet was the key to the Liu inheritance which would be, of course, the land and maybe some type of precious coins or jewels.

Liu smiled inwardly as he took the amulet. Memories flashed through his mind as he recalled the day his father told him about how a large golden amulet had been fashioned by the local blacksmith.

Engraved on the front of the amulet was the Yin Yang symbol, surrounded by the Chinese characters for the Five Elements: Metal, Water, Wood, Fire, and Earth. Surrounding both were the eight Kua from the I Ching. This pattern represented the major concepts in Chinese philosophy. Even though Liu's father only practiced the family martial arts, the design of Yin Yang, the Five Elements, and the eight Kua also represented the martial arts of Tai Chi Chuan, Hsing-Yi Chuan, and Pa Kua Chang.

On the backside of the amulet were Chinese characters from Buddhist, Taoist, and Confucian philosophies. Looking at only one part of the amulet, the characters seemed to be random words, but looking at the whole backside of the amulet, the order of the characters gave each meaning.

His father had related how the blacksmith had found it interesting that the amulet was made out of pure gold. The blacksmith could neither read nor write, so he didn't know what the characters meant. He'd been instructed to cut the amulet into four pieces so the amulet could only be put together again if each of the four pieces was present. One piece was the key to all the others and whoever had that piece could control not only the wealth of the Liu family but also the wealth of the information on the scrolls Liu always carried with him.

The four pieces had to fit together in a certain order for the front and back to make sense. This was done so no one person could guess what the other three pieces looked like or what the inscription said.

The blacksmith was further instructed to cover the gold with another metal to hide the gold and then drill a hole at the edge of each of the four pieces so it could be hung from the neck by a string.

Liu remembered the instructions his father gave him concerning the four pieces of the amulet. One was to be held by the oldest male child, another was to go to the family of the faithful servant who had served the Liu family for generations, another was to go the temple for safe keeping, and the last—and most important—piece went to Liu for safe keeping. Liu had memorized the inscriptions on each amulet. This was another way of making sure whomever had an amulet had an original and not a forgery. The Abbot at the temple also knew the characters and how to match up the coins. What he did not know was the meaning behind the characters, the order of the characters, and how it all related to the information Liu possessed. The information on the amulets was the key to deciphering the information on the scrolls. Without that critical key, the information on the scrolls was not anywhere near as valuable as it would be with the key.

Liu turned the amulet over to make sure none of the gold was showing through the covering metal. He was pleased to see the amulet had not been tampered with. He was more pleased when Pei Ke, without hesitancy, gave back the amulet. He knew the monk had told Pei Ke the history of the amulet and value of what he held in his possession.

"Pei Ke, I want you to continue to hold on to the amulet. I gave it to you for a reason. It is yours. You have been told that it is a key to a great fortune, but you do not as yet understand the significance or extent of that fortune. At the appropriate time, I will share the information with you. Remember to always safeguard it with your life."

Pei Ke was thankful he had not relinquished the amulet to the Abbot. When Liu had left him with the Abbot, he'd had to make a decision as to whether or not to give the amulet to the Abbot. Even though his mind was in great turmoil, he knew his decision to follow Liu had been correct. He didn't know if he had arrived at the decision because of his own intuition, the influence of the Abbot, or the guidance of the goddess Kuan Yin. Perhaps it had been the Universal Energy Liu was always talking about. He didn't really care.

# CHAPTER THIRTY-FOUR

Master, as we walk, may I ask you some questions about Chinese martial arts? I would like to know as much as possible. You've told me about Pa Kua Chang and its founder Tong Hai Chuan, Hsing-Yi Chuan and its founder Yue Fe, and Tai Chi Chuan and its founder Chang San Fang.

"You have mentioned other martial arts such as Choi Le Fut, Praying Mantis, and Hung Gar. And of course, you've mentioned you have studied Shaolin and your family's martial arts. What do I need to know about these other martial arts?"

"There is much information about Chinese martial arts for you to learn," said Liu. "The history is extensive and there are conflicting stories about how each of the hundred or so martial arts began. What I am going to tell you is what has been passed on to me by other martial artists and what I have read in the ancient manuscripts.

"It is agreed by many historians, that one of the oldest Chinese martial arts is Shuai Jiao. Some say it is over four thousand years old. Others say three thousand years old. The interesting thing about Shuai Jiao is how it has remained with us for so long. The art distinguishes itself from other Chinese martial arts in that it is a grappling or wrestling art with numerous throws and joint locks. For close-in fighting, it is probably one of best martial arts to know and practice. It is quite simple, but brutal in its effectiveness. I have watched individuals practice this art and am always amazed at the superior conditioning necessary to take the repeated throws and take downs characteristic of this system. One should definitely learn it at a young age because the human body needs the conditioning early in life to withstand the constant impact with the ground."

"I imagine those who practice the art need to be incredibly strong to lift people up and throw them to the ground," said Pei Ke.

"Strength is important, but the most important factors are balance and leverage. The practitioner uses his balance and the unbalanced position of his opponent to make the art effective."

"Master, do you know Shuai Jiao?"

"No, I did not have the opportunity to learn it. It is not possible to learn all the arts. It takes a good part of one's lifetime to be a master of any of these arts. It is often knowing the right person or being in the right place at the right time that leads to the opportunity of finding a good teacher. I can't stress enough the importance of finding a good teacher. There are many out there professing to know martial arts, but many are either lying or simply cannot teach well what they know."

Pei Ke reflected on how lucky he was to be at the right place at the right time. In the short couple of years he had known Liu, he had seen the master attacked numerous times, and always come out victorious.

"Master, if you had the opportunity to study Shuai Jiao now, would you take advantage of it?"

"At this stage in my life, I am too old to take on another art. Any martial art is a lifetime of study. The more you practice and study the art, the more you gain an insight into the esoteric factors of the art. Anyone who says he is a master of a martial art after only a brief study is not only fooling himself but is also doing a tremendous disservice to those he teaches.

"The Chinese martial arts I already know provide me with what I need. I know you feel I am a master of these arts. It is true I have studied them for many years, but what you don't know is that as I continue to practice and research these arts, I gain a deeper understanding of them from not only a physical perspective but also from a philosophical and mental one. In addition, I gain an understanding of the energy associated with each of these arts. The energy aspect and how to use it in self defense has always intrigued me. I have enough to learn to keep me busy forever.

"To answer your question about other Chinese martial arts would take many days. However, let me give you an additional insight into the development of Chinese martial arts.

"Other than Shuai Jiao, almost all Chinese martial arts can trace their development in one aspect or another to the Shaolin Temple in Henan Province. The name 'Shaolin' means 'little forest,' but here it refers to the temple.

"The martial art got its start at the temple when the monk Bodhidharma brought Zen Buddhism to China from India. He settled at the temple. In teaching his subjects Buddhism, he developed exercises to keep them healthy. These exercises were the foundation for the martial art of Shaolin. If we are ever in the area, I will take you to the temple."

"Master, can we go when we are finished in Beijing?"

"I don't know when I will be finished in Beijing. What you need to do now is to concentrate and review what you have already learned."

# CHAPTER THIRTY-FIVE

"Master, do all people recover from illness at the same rate? I guess I am asking if all people need the same number of treatments."

"There are a number of different factors determining recovery times. It depends on both the patient and the doctor.

"For the patient, it depends on how carefully he or she follows the directions of the doctor in taking the herbal formulas as indicated, and whether the patient returns for the recommended number of follow up visits. You have to think of acupuncture as a process of therapy rather than a single-visit solution. It is the responsibility of the doctor to explain this to the patient and to impress on the patient the importance of the follow-up visits. It is the responsibility of the patient to follow the doctor's recommendation."

Pei Ke thought for a moment before commenting.

"In other words," said Pei Ke, "the doctor and the patient work as a team. It is not the patient seeing the doctor or the doctor seeing the patient. It is a team effort."

"Yes, it is a team effort with a clear objective and a means to solve a problem."

"So the patient is just as important as the doctor in solving these health care issues."

"Yes, of course," said Liu.

"It is now important to know the doctor's role in why some patients get better and heal faster than others. It comes down to the diagnosis and the treatment. If the diagnosis is wrong, then the treatment is going to be wrong. The diagnosis can be correct but the treatment can be wrong. Seldom, if ever, is the diagnosis wrong and the treatment correct. Such a situation would indicate a very incompetent doctor.

"If the diagnosis is partially correct than the treatment is going to be partially correct. A good example is when the doctor treats the symptoms, which are like the branches of the problem, rather than treating the root of the problem.

"The doctor can continue treating the branches and eventually the patient will see an improvement, which may or may not last. It would be better if the diagnosis was correct from the start. Then the doctor could treat the root of the problem, which will give far superior results for the patient.

"Some doctors knowingly treat the branches of the problem, even after they've determined the root. That way, they force the patient to return to them again and again when the lesser treatments wear off.

"It is more ethical to immediately identify and treat the root of the problem. Very few patients want to take herbal prescriptions that only cover up the problem. Treating the root saves the patient time and money."

"Master, can you give me more information on this branch and root concept? As you explain branch and root, it sounds like a large tree where the symptoms are the limbs of the tree and the cause is the root of the tree."

"That is one way to explain it. I think of it as a situation where some of the branches and leaves of the tree don't look right. They may be diseased, misshapen, discolored, or stunted. I can cut off those branches or leaves and then the tree will look nice. Of course, if I cut off too much or cut it off in an unbalanced or unnatural way, then the tree doesn't look aesthetically pleasing. And sooner or later, more leaves and branches will start looking bad because I haven't really solved the problem.

"On the other hand, I can find out why the tree has the problem. Once I find out why it has the problem I can work from the inside with the proper nutrition or treatments to help it grow. Once the internal problem is fixed, the external problem will be fixed. Trying to solve the internal problem by continuing to change or cover up the external problem does not solve the overall problem. In many instances, the problem will only keep getting worse. You can see this when people move from one area of China to another and find they have allergies they never had before. Of course, we can cover up the symptoms, but why not solve the problem with acupuncture and herbal formulas so the symptoms go away?

"Another example would be skin problems such as acne. We can put an herbal paste on the skin to reduce the irritation, but this may not solve the underlying problem. The problem is internal and not external. The external skin problem is only a manifestation of the internal problem. We need to solve the internal or root of the problem."

"Master, how long does it take to be able to distinguish between the branch and the root of a problem?"

"It depends on your ability and study. Many are able to distinguish simple problems quite easily with just a little study. It is the complex health care issues, where the signs and symptoms blend into more than one category that pose a challenge to us to be able to come up with an appropriate diagnosis."

"Master, have you ever had a situation where you could not come up with a diagnosis?"

Liu thought for a minute before answering the question.

"I can usually come up with a diagnosis, but there have been instances when the diagnosis has been difficult because of conflicting symptoms. This is especially true if the patient has multiple problems. In these situations, it is clinical experience and not book learning that is important. Everyone who has ever been in any form of health care knows this to be true. It is important for you as the doctor to constantly study and research so that you are able to give the patient the best possible care.

"There is one thing that I would like to mention. I wanted to mention this to you before. Now is a good opportunity. There is nothing wrong with the patient going to another doctor for a second opinion if the patient feels the doctor is not giving the type of treatment he should receive.

"The patient has hired the doctor. The doctor has not hired the patient. There are different levels of competence with doctors, but as a doctor you want to provide the best care so the patients do not feel they have to go somewhere else. Do you understand?"

"Yes, Master."

# CHAPTER THIRTY-SIX

Master, I watch you do Tai Chi Chuan and it looks so beautiful. When you use it as a martial art your movements are so fast and controlled. What is your secret? What do I need to know to be as good as you?"

"Over the years, Tai Chi Chuan practitioners have discovered a number of principles that help them to be effective in the art. Tai Chi Chuan can be practiced a number of different ways. As is often the case, what I am about to share with you is only my opinion. Some would agree, but others would surely disagree with me.

"First, Tai Chi Chuan can be practiced with the intent of using the moves as self defense. As you do each move, you visualize an opponent and you imagine using the movements for self defense. When you do this, you need to think about where your body is in relation to your opponent. You need to also visualize where you are touching, grabbing, and holding the opponent. There are many movements in Tai Chi Chuan where Chin Na applications are part of the movement. This is especially true of the Tai Chi Chuan I teach. If you want to be effective in real life situations, you must know these movements and mentally do the Chin Na applications as you move through the form.

"Second, I agree with the old masters who espouse slow continuous practice of Tai Chi Chuan to develop ones internal energy. Some of the old masters were quite adept at Tai Chi Chuan, and it is due to the way they have cultivated their Qi.

"As you do the moves, you must feel the energy in your body and it should flow from one move to another. Many students indicate they feel the energy only in certain moves. It seems to be blocked as they move into the next posture. This problem can be caused by a misalignment of the body, especially the hips and shoulders.

"Third, the movements can be done in static positions. Each move is executed normally and then held for a few seconds before moving on to the next position. This is like doing Qi Gong but it is Tai Chi Chuan. I feel this helps the energy to catch up with the movement. Many disagree with me, but my experience tells me it is effective. When I teach you Tai Chi Chuan, you will see what I mean, especially after you have developed your Qi Gong abilities. In essence, the Tai Chi Chuan becomes one form of Qi Gong.

"Fourth, Tai Chi Chuan can be done fast. It is one thing to do it slowly to develop the correct manner of executing each of the many postures. It is another to be able to do the movements very fast. You will need to do them very fast if you are ever going to use them as a martial art.

"Fifth, to be really good at Tai Chi Chuan as a martial art you need to have a partner you can use to help you with the dynamics of each move. Even though you may know the application of each move, there are subtleties of each move you will only discover when you have a partner. The partner will help you learn the intricacies of each of the moves and experience how weight shifts, rooting, and balance are crucial in the effective utilization of the movements.

"Sixth, you need to do push hands, which is an advanced two-person, controlled set of movements. This practice will help you enhance your balance and feel where the force is coming from when you have an opponent. Actually, push hands can be quite fun if it is approached with the right attitude. As a beginning student, it is not trying to always win over your opponent by constantly unbalancing him, but helping him to know how to react to the force of the energy as it is applied to different parts of the body. In turn, you will understand how to use your body with the minimum amount of force to accomplish the maximum amount of directed leverage."

"Which one of these methods of doing Tai Chi Chuan do you prefer?"

"I do them all. In addition, not only will I do the form in the precise order the movements were taught, but I will improvise and do the movements out of sequence. In this way I am not conditioned to always do one move followed by another. I might do the movement of Snake Creeps Down followed by Golden Chicken Stands on one Leg one day, but the following day I might do Snake Creeps Down followed Fair Lady Throws the Shuttle. When I do this, the form never looks the same, but the benefit is still there, and I am training myself for realistic combat situations."

"Master, will you show me push hands?"

"You have not learned Tai Chi Chuan yet."

"I know, but if it is fun, I would like to try it with you."

"Very well. Stand with your feet shoulder width apart and your toes straight ahead. Shift the weight to your right foot and turn on the heel of your left foot approximately forty-five degrees to the left. Bend both legs and shift your weight to your left foot. Now put your right foot forward. Shift your weight forward so you feel balanced."

"How far do I step forwards?"

Liu adjusted Pei Ke's stance, moving his legs and feet to be appropriate for his height and shoulder width. Liu took up a position that was the mirror image of Pei Ke with his right foot alongside Pei Ke's separated by about a foot. Both were in exactly the same position facing each other.

"I want you to put both of your hands on my chest and push against my chest."

Pei Ke lifted his hands and placed them on Liu's chest and looked at his master.

"Push," said Liu.

Pei Ke pushed against Liu's chest, but nothing happened. Liu did not move.

"Harder," said Liu.

Pei Ke pushed harder, but Liu still did not move. It seemed strange to Pei Ke. He was pushing hard but Liu wasn't doing anything. Liu remained soft with no resistance, but he was completely immobile.

"Harder," said Liu. "Push as hard as you can."

Pei Ke adjusted his hands on Liu's chest and pushed as hard as he could. Nothing happened. Liu was totally relaxed with no visible signs of tension or force, yet Pei Ke could not move him. Liu was not leaning forward into the push nor was he tightening his muscles to resist the force. To Pei Ke it seemed as if there was an immovable wall and the more he pushed, the more the wall resisted, but it resisted with no force.

"Push harder," said Liu.

Pei Ke pushed with everything he had. He still couldn't move Liu. Liu turned his waist slightly to the right and Pei Ke fell forward and tumbled to the ground.

"Master, how did you do that? As I was pushing against your chest all of a sudden there was nothing to push against. It seems you just dissolved the entire force of my push."

"Actually," said Liu, "I used your own force to defeat you. Let's try again."

Liu and Pei Ke did the same scenario a couple of times. Pei Ke would push as hard as he could. Liu would redirect the force; and Pei Ke would become unbalanced to the point where he would stumble or fall.

"Pei Ke, place your hands on my chest again and slightly push."

It felt entirely different. Before there was a solid wall that was totally immovable. Now there was nothing to push against. It felt like he was pushing against a round ball that was always moving.

"Pei Ke, I want you to use varying degrees of force and push against my chest. You can use a lot of force or just a little force, but I want you to push me over."

Pei Ke did as he was instructed by Liu. No matter how he pushed, there was nothing to push against. He tried pushing more with one hand than the other. He tried pushing downwards and upwards, but there was still nothing to push against. The faster he pushed, the more unbalanced he became. He tried not pushing and then immediately pushing very hard. It was all to no avail. He could not push Liu because he could not find a solid point to push against. Everything he touched had no center to push against. Liu became a ball with no center.

As Pei Ke was pushing, Liu changed his focus and Pei Ke sensed finally he had something to push against and he pushed as hard as he could push. Nothing happened. It was just like before when he'd tried to push against the immovable wall. Again Liu did not move, nor did he exert any effort to resist Pei Ke's push.

"Pei Ke, you have now been pushing for over twenty minutes and you have yet to unbalance me. You have expended a lot of energy to no avail.

Now let's reverse the situation. I want you to stay in this same position. I am going to push against you, and I want you to prevent me from unbalancing you. Let me know when you are ready."

"Master, I am ready."

As soon as the words were out of his mouth Pei Ke was off balance and thrown to the ground. He got up and placed himself in the push hands position. No matter how hard he tried, he could not resist the force Liu was applying to him. The strange thing was that Liu wasn't exerting any strength. Pei Ke expected to feel a lot of force, but he felt nothing in comparison to what happened to him when Liu had touched him. It was so fast he could barely comprehend what had happened. He had been pushed forward and backward, and he had no control of how he was being pushed or in what direction he was being pushed.

"Master, how do you do that? It's really amazing. No matter how hard I push against you there is no way I am going to push you over. No matter how hard I resist there is no way I can prevent you from pushing me over. There has to be a trick to it, and I'd really like to learn it."

"There is no trick to push hands. It is a skill most can learn, but it takes years of dedicated practice to be able to do it, and you need to study with someone who can teach you correctly. If you don't learn correctly you will only acquire a limited degree of skill, and it won't be enough for you to use it on the street. I was fortunate to learn from some of the best and I will pass the skills on to you at the appropriate time."

"Master, I am going to guess there are certain principles I need to know."

"Everything I teach has principles. Those who accept the principles readily, learn the fastest. Those who want to shorten the learning cycle or circumvent the principles only end up frustrated when they can't do it right."

"Master, as you know I am willing to learn the correct way and to do it like it is supposed to be done."

"You also want to learn Pa Kua Chang and Hsing-Yi Chuan. How are you going to learn them all plus, Qi Gong, weapons, Chin Na, and Traditional Chinese Medicine?"

Without thinking Pei Ke blurted out. "I guess I'll be studying with you for many years." As soon as he had said it, he realized the commitment it would take and how his life would be tied to Liu. Liu could see the doubt in Pei Ke's face.

"Think about it," said Liu.

He wondered what he should do and whether or not he should talk with Liu and get his advice about this life long study program. Liu would not be around forever and there was a good possibility that he would not be able to learn everything Liu knew. These and some other questions went through Pei Ke's mind as they continued their walk towards Beijing.

Liu sensed there was something on Pei Ke's mind, but he wanted his student to ask. The Universal Energy would give Pei Ke the right direction in life.

Liu turned his thoughts to the time when he was a child growing up under the tutelage of his father and mother. He remembered his father teaching him strength-building exercises. His training started when he was six years old. At first his father guided him in exercises such as horse stance practice, where his feet were spread apart one and a half times the distance of the width of his shoulders. He would sit in a semi-crouched position with his knees bent. In this position, it was natural for the weight of the body to shift forward so the knees protruded past the toes. His father corrected this tendency and Liu had to sit with his knees over his toes—but not protruding past his toes. At first Liu hated the horse stance. He had the feeling he was going to fall backwards. The pain and discomfort in his legs were almost unbearable.

Initially, he could only stay bent in the horse stance position for a few minutes. As his hips and back opened up, through the stretching of the muscles, he found he could bear up under the discomfort and sit in the position almost indefinitely. The horse stance training had been an everyday routine, except for one day a week when Liu was allowed to rest.

After his legs became stronger, his father would position his arms and shoulders so a pole or staff could be placed on them and not fall off. His father would do the same thing. With both of them in a horse stance his father would instruct him in the various tenets of martial arts, especially the family martial arts.

Liu remembered the first fight he had as a child. Normally the family was a self contained unit, hidden away in their valley, but on some weekends and special occasions, his father and sometimes the whole family would trek to the nearest village to stock up on needed supplies. His father wanted the family to know what it was like to be outside the valley, and for the villagers not to think of the Liu family as being isolated.

Liu's father had numerous acquaintances in the village and was considered one of the elders, even though they did not live in the village. On many occasions, his father would be consulted on village matters. Liu's father was the main benefactor in bringing monks to the village and was responsible for donating a significant amount of money for construction of the temple.

When Liu was about twelve years old, he was on one of these trips to the village. His father wanted to visit one of the local artisans to commission some work. Liu was given the run of the village and told to be back in an hour. Liu had liked the opportunity to walk around the village and see the various vendors and the wares they had to offer. He didn't know anyone his age and barely knew his father's acquaintances.

Every community of any size has one or more individuals who are always in trouble. This village was no exception. It wasn't more than ten minutes after leaving his father that he rounded a corner and inadvertently bumped into a boy carrying metal cups of soy bean milk. The liquid spilled all over the boy.

Liu was very apologetic for the unfortunate accident and even offered to pay for the spilt soy milk. The boy yelled and pushed Liu to the ground. Liu got up and was pushed against the wall. The boy held Liu to the wall. Liu continued to be apologetic and even though he had no money on him, offered to pay for new clothes.

The more Liu spoke, the angrier the boy became. Liu started to struggle and the boy hit him in the face. Liu remembered the fear and paralysis that overwhelmed him to inaction. He soon realized that while the boy who'd hit him was about his age, he was much stockier and taller than him.

He knew he should defend himself but, even though he had studied martial arts from his father since he was six years old, he had never been in an actual fight. His training had always been in a controlled environment, even with his brothers. He had never hit someone in anger, and so he hesitated.

The beating became more intense as Liu recovered from his fright and started to fight back. Every move Liu made in self defense, the boy countered and hit harder. Liu was taking a hard beating when the boy was yanked off his feet and thrown to the ground.

Liu saw his father standing next to the boy. The boy threw a punch at Liu's father, but the punch dissolved into thin air as Liu's father sidestepped it. The boy, sensing he was at a disadvantage, ran down the alley.

Liu's father never said a word about the altercation. The walk back to their valley was done in silence, but the next morning before the sun rose, Liu's father had him up and training in the family's ancient martial arts. The training from that day forward took on a totally different direction. It was no longer a mastery of conditioning and forms practice, but actual applications and the various concepts needed to win a fight. Liu was later thankful for that initial beating and the harsh training that followed, for it opened the door for him to be able to master Chinese martial arts.

"Master, is it appropriate for me to ask you a question? You have been quiet for over an hour."

"Pei Ke, I have been deep in thought. Yes, ask me a question."

"When you treat patients, you ask the patients about their health. What the patient tells you, leads you to make a decision about which meridian and which acupuncture point to use."

"Give me an example," said Liu.

"If the patient says they have an upset stomach, then you would use an acupuncture point on the Stomach Meridian."

"Yes, what the patient tells me helps me to make a decision."

"Then it would be easy for us to decide in our treatment plan to always use the meridian associated with the complaint."

"It would be one piece of information to help you. The question you need to ask yourself is what to do if the patient has a headache. There is no such thing as a headache meridian. There are however, meridians to treat headaches. The question is which meridian to use. This is where the differential diagnosis is important."

Pei Ke thought for a few minutes. Liu was going to add some additional information, but decided to wait for Pei Ke to ask the next question.

"Master, can I ask some questions about Tai Chi Chuan?

"Pei Ke, your mind is again wandering. Let's stay with the topic.

"As you know there are twelve meridians in the body and each is associated with a particular organ. Each organ has a certain function in the body. So in our differential diagnosis, we can assume a dysfunction of an organ will lead to a specific complaint by the patient. As an example, if the patient has a stomachache, then the Stomach Meridian may be a good choice for treating the patient. Another possibility is that the area of the body on which a particular symptom is found may be the clue to which meridian to use.

"Let's use a headache as an example. As I just mentioned, there is no headache meridian. However, there are meridians that affect different areas of the head. When the patient has a headache on the side of the head, then I know it could be the Gallbladder Meridian because the path that this meridian follows is on the side of the head.

"If the patient complains of a sore throat, difficulty in breathing, and a cough which meridian would you suspect?"

"Master, I would suspect it would be the Lung Meridian."

"You are correct. But the Lung Meridian would also be able to treat neck pain and chest pain because the meridian passes through those areas. Since the Stomach Meridian, Large Intestine Meridian, and the Gall Bladder Meridian pass through the area, you could also use those meridians. Your refinement in asking questions, plus the other tools you have learned about diagnosis, will help you to isolate which meridian or meridians are the ones you need to use."

Pei Ke thought for a few minutes trying to come up with examples in his mind.

"Master, then there are certain manifestations associated with each one of the meridians."

"Yes, that is correct," said Liu. "Your ability to diagnosis will depend, in part, on your questioning ability. This questioning ability will depend on your past clinical experience as you become more familiar with clinical manifestations. Each of the meridians has a specific set of manifestations for you to remember. There are additional symptoms for the Lung Meridian. They include pain along the inside of the arm, wrist and thumb pain, elbow pain, and restricted range of motion in the neck."

"Master, you have given me the manifestations for the Lung Meridian. What are the manifestations for the rest of the meridians?"

"Pei Ke, we have had discussions about the heart before. What would you think would be the manifestations for the Heart Meridian?"

Pei Ke thought for a few moments.

"If the heart is involved, I would suspect there would be some type of irregular heartbeat, chest pain in the heart area, and problems along the Heart Meridian. Am I correct?"

"Yes, you are correct. Many practitioners will not agree with what I am going to tell you, but from generations of clinical experience doctors have discovered that when there is a problem with the heart energy, the patient can also have insomnia, night sweats, hot and sweaty palms, thirst, emotional problems, problems on the face and mouth, and lack of taste. Remember we had a discussion about your mother and her problems? So it is important to know these manifestations in your diagnosis process. I will cover the other meridians and their manifestations at another time. Just remember what you have learned today."

# CHAPTER THIRTY-SEVEN

"Master, you have explained the concept of Qi in our bodies more than once, but it is a difficult concept for me to understand. It seems that each time you explain something to me you explain it a little bit differently. Would you explain Qi to me one more time?"

"Yes, it is a difficult concept to understand. The more you become familiar with the concept and how it affects our bodies, the easier it is for you to grasp all of its implications.

"Basically, we have energy in our bodies. This energy is what keeps us alive. If you feel your pulse, you will feel your heart beat. The heart beats because there is energy keeping it beating. This energy comes from the food we eat, the liquids we drink, and the exercise we do, especially if it is Qi Gong exercise or Tai Chi Chuan. When we eat, a transformation process converts the food we eat into energy. This energy is then circulated throughout our bodies.

"As you know, the energy is circular in motion, meaning it flows from one part of our body to another through the meridian system. As I have explained before, the energy flows from lung to large intestine to stomach and continues through the rest of our bodies through the meridian system. The way the ancient Chinese described this flow of the energy going from one meridian to another implied there is lung Qi and large intestine Qi.

"Well, we know there is only one Qi, but it manifests itself in different ways. This is the case when the lung energy in the Lung Meridian passes to the Large Intestine Meridian. The large intestine energy takes on a different quality than that which is present in the Lung Meridian. It is all the same energy, but it takes on different qualities or essences as it brings energy to its specific organ.

"Thus, we have lung energy for the Lung Meridian and large intestine energy for the Large Intestine Meridian. Again, the energy is the same, but its essence takes on different qualities.

"Does that help you understand the concept of Qi?"

"Yes, it helps, and I remember this explanation of yours before, but it still doesn't answer some of the more complex questions. For example, in the past we discussed Liver Fire Rising as a condition that can cause migraines. If we solve the problem of Liver Fire Rising, then the migraines will go away. And as I understand it, we are not covering up the problem or providing some kind of temporary relief, but we're actually providing a resolution to the problem. Solve the Liver Fire Rising and the headaches go away permanently. I assume Liver Fire Rising is a Qi problem. Am I correct?"

"Yes, you are correct. It is an imbalance in the Qi causing the problem."

"Since it is an imbalance in the Qi, what or how has the Qi changed?"

"It is the quality of the Qi that has changed. As an example, suppose you have a fresh apple. It tastes one way when you eat it. If you leave the apple in the sun for an extended period of time you will still have an apple, but the quality of the apple has changed because of the heat. The same is with Qi; the quality can change.

"In Liver Fire Rising the quality of the liver energy has changed, or the liver energy has become blocked, and that is what causes the migraine. When the energy is restored to what it is supposed to be, the migraine will go away. It is the responsibility of the acupuncturist to discern what the change has been. In other words there are many possible liver energy qualities that differ from the norm. The signs and symptoms will tell the practitioner about the quality of the change.

"Through thousands of years of experience, we have determined that if there is an aberration in the quality of the liver Qi, then there are certain points that can be used to treat the problem. For this reason Liver Fire Rising and Liver Blood Deficiency are each treated differently.

"When the quality of the Qi in the Liver Meridian changes, it is different from the changing quality of the Qi in another meridian. Each meridian has its own essence of Qi. For example, if the Qi of the Liver Meridian becomes excess, then there will be a certain reaction in the body. If the Qi of another meridian is excess, then there will be a totally different reaction. Remember, the Qi of each meridian is the same, but it takes on a different essence when it passes from one meridian to another. Many of the signs and symptoms of each condition will be the same for each patient."

"In other words," said Pei Ke, "everyone will have the same symptoms, and that is how we are able to diagnose the problem."

"It is better to say the signs and symptoms are a broad category and people with the same condition may have many of the same symptoms."

"Why don't they have all the same symptoms?"

"The reason is because of our constitutional backgrounds. A patient's parents, grandparents, great grandparents, and so forth gave them their physical and emotional makeup. If we compare the constitutions of two people who have excess liver Qi, we might see a slightly different combination of problems. That is why with Liver Fire Rising, one patient may have ringing in the ears and another would not."

"In other words," said Pei Ke. "There is a large grouping of symptoms for Liver Fire Rising and the patient may have one or more of those symptoms, but it is highly unlikely if you had three or four patients they would all have exactly the same symptoms."

"That is correct," said Liu.

"That seems to help me understand Qi a little better."

"I know it is difficult to understand. It has been difficult for everyone who studies these arts."

"Master, what other concepts do I need to know to be a competent doctor?"

"You will need to know more than what you already know. You will find the more you know the more you need to know to be very competent in this profession. Too many practitioners feel they have mastered this beautiful art. In essence, you never master the art. You only get better and better over time as clinical experience opens the doors to new treatment protocols.

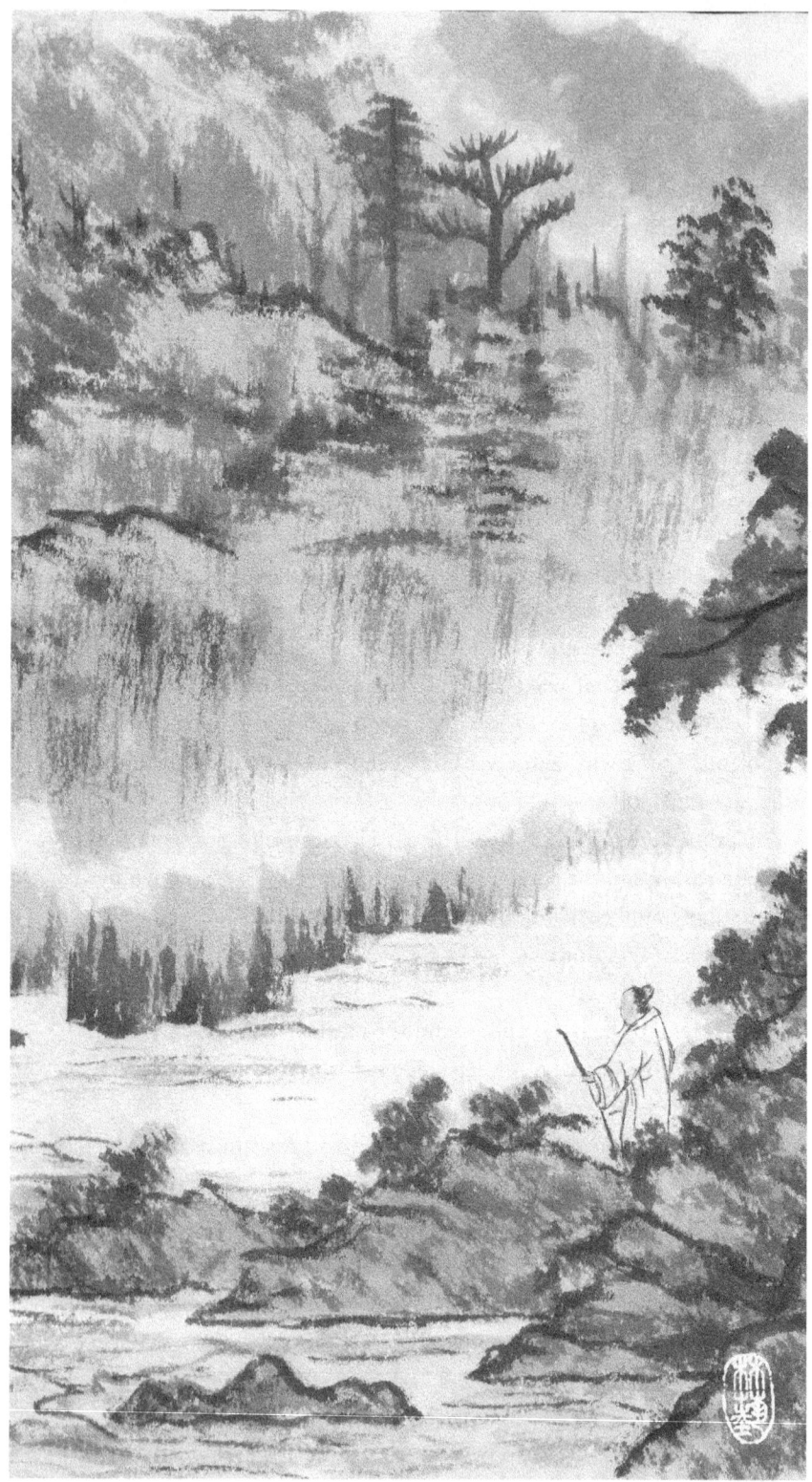

# CHAPTER THIRTY-EIGHT

The early morning darkness gave way to the first light of dawn as snowflakes fell on the road. They had experienced snow before on this journey, but had been lucky to not have a lot of accumulation. What snow did fall often melted as the temperature rose during the day.

On this particular day, they were no more than a day's journey from their destination. The terrain was still mostly farm land, but there were more houses than before. The plots of land were not as large as when they were in more rural areas. The quality of the construction of the houses was different. It had even changed from what they'd seen the previous day. Liu suspected the sophistication of the farmers was different from what they had experienced since leaving his ancestral home.

About two hours before sunset, they came upon a large village. The size of the village warranted a Buddhist temple. The local inhabitants almost always wanted to be able to worship as their parents and grandparents had done for generations.

As they entered the village, there were only a few shops that remained open. Most of the transactions for the day had been consummated earlier and the approaching evening meant everyone needed to close up for the day. However, there was one shop that had not closed, and it stood out from the others. Liu was intrigued that the shop remained open. He looked at the building, studying something about its construction.

230 • Richard A. Peck

"This building is laid out quite uniquely," said Liu. "The angle is not the same as it is with the rest of the buildings. Look at the sign on the building."

Pei Ke looked at the sign and smiled. It was a fortune teller and Liu was going in. Pei Ke had had his fortune told before and in some cases, what was told to him had been accurate. In other cases, he felt the fortune teller was just making things up. He didn't know whether to believe it or not.

As they entered the shop, Liu stopped quickly and Pei Ke almost bumped into him.

"Pei Ke, this place has unsettled energy and we may not want to spend too much time here. In fact, we should go now."

As Liu turned to leave, Liu heard the noise of a sword being pulled out of a scabbard. He turned just in time to see an elderly man with a sword standing in the middle of the shop.

"If you are here to rob me, I will slice you up before you take two more steps," said the man.

"We are not here to rob you. We are traveling through and we saw your shop and thought you were open. We will be leaving now."

"I was told to watch out for you. You fit the description perfectly. They said an elderly monk and a younger man may stop. They said you've killed and robbed many in the previous towns."

"Who said this?" demanded Liu.

"Those kind men who came through here earlier this morning told me about you. Of course, I did not believe them, but I now know they were telling the truth."

"I assure you," said Liu. "We are not criminals and we mean you no harm. We are leaving now and will not bother you."

Liu turned, opened the door, and gently pushed Pei Ke out.

"Master, do you think those men that have attacked us had anything to do with this?"

"Probably," said Liu. "Let's put some distance between us and this shop."

# CHAPTER THIRTY-NINE

Liu and Pei Ke continued on their journey, distancing themselves from the encounter in the shop. Liu knew they were probably being followed, but felt comfortable nonetheless.

It had been many years since he had last been in what he called the city of mystery. There were so many things to do in Beijing. He could meet with his former friends and catch up on what had taken place since he had last been there, or he could visit one of the temples he'd frequented in the past. They would be willing to give him food and lodging during his stay.

What puzzled him was the sheer number of people in the city who were there to satisfy the needs of the emperor. He was sure the emperor, who was secluded behind the walls of the Forbidden City, never realized the extent of what was done for him or to him.

Eunuchs and administrative officials had absolute control over the emperor's daily activities. Liu wondered who was worse off, the eunuchs or the administrative officials. The emperor was secluded behind the walls of the city. Liu wondered if in reality, it was forbidden for the people to enter the city, or was it forbidden for the emperor to visit with those who he ruled? Liu felt it was a mystery reserved for those who dealt in mysteries.

As they entered the city, Liu realized the city hadn't changed much since he was last there. The familiar sights, sounds, and smells were as he had remembered.

The strong Beijing accent was a little hard to get used to at first. Typically, the Chinese language had four tones to differentiate words. This was true in Beijing as well, but there was a distinct heavy 'r' sound at the end of some words making the Chinese language spoken in Beijing difficult to understand. It would take both of them a couple of days to get accustomed to the accent.

He needed to be sure he didn't stand out too much as being from the countryside. There was always someone trying to take advantage of unsuspecting visitors.

They entered the city from the West Gate. It was a massive structure designed to guard the city from invaders. Pei Ke had never seen a gate of such enormity and decorated with such intricate stone work in his whole life. Finally inside the city, they headed for Nan Luo Gu Street.

Liu was familiar with this area, having visited with some friends many years previous. In fact, ten years earlier he had stayed with a well-known individual in this same area. It was in this area he would try to reestablish old acquaintances. He didn't know if his old acquaintances wanted to see him, but he would at least make an effort.

That night they stayed at one of the local temples.

# CHAPTER FORTY

The following morning, Liu and Pei Ke rose early and took breakfast with the monks in the temple. They were both excited to finally be away from the countryside. Liu looked forward to revisiting and rekindling old memories. Pei Ke was excited about all the new sights and sounds he was to experience.

After breakfast they had a quick conversation with the Abbot of the temple. Once outside the walls of the temple, they walked toward some shops Liu had known when he lived in the city. The cleaning crews were out early picking up the garbage from the previous day. The little shops with the morning delicacies were already open and they could smell the cooking oil and hot soybean drink being prepared for the morning crowds.

This was Liu's favorite time of the day. It was the beginning of something new just like the Tao which was in continuous motion, evolving from one phase to another phase, always returning to the original. The cycle continued forever just as the morning sun had risen in the East since the beginning of time.

To Liu, it was like a rebirth each and every day. It was a new start, always invigorating him. He knew from what he had been taught and from his many years of experience, that the practice of Qi Gong and Tai Chi Chuan in the morning was the foundation for keeping one healthy for many years.

234 • Richard A. Peck

They walked past an area where there were various street shops and vendors.

"Master, look at the jade pendants for sale. They must be very expensive. I remember seeing jade and porcelain at Mr. Wang's house."

"Do you know the history of jade?" asked Liu.

Pei Ke turned to the shop keeper. He was about to ask him some questions when Liu asked. "Do you make these jade pieces?"

"I don't make them myself," said the shop keeper. "They are made by my father and grandfather. The family tradition has been passed on for generations. I am studying from them now. They are both away from the shop but will be back later."

"Do you know the history of jade and why it is valued in Chinese culture?" asked Liu.

"Yes, I do. Jade is highly valued in our culture, and has played a significant social role over the generations. According to my grandfather, the discovery and use of jade goes back almost eight thousand years. Initially, jade was thought to be a gift from the gods and was used for decorative purposes. Women would wear round jade earrings. There would be a small slit in the oval or round earring so the earring could be slid over the ear lobe.

"Later jade was used for practical things like tool making, utensils, and dinner ware. As our culture developed, so did the use of jade. It was quite often part of burial ceremonies. Jade carvings were placed in the grave in the belief the jade would make the body and soul immortal in the afterlife.

"As we developed socially and economically, the various emperors began to cherish jade for themselves. The artisans would create specific bowls and utensils for royal use. The value of the jade increased and various dictates came about concerning its use and ownership. As you can imagine, jade became a symbol of power, status, and wealth. Gentleman would wear a jade amulet around their neck as a sign of virtue."

"Where does jade come from?" asked Pei Ke.

The shop keeper smiled, happy to have a chance to show off what he knew.

"Jade was first discovered by ancient people living in the northeast. Today we get it from different areas of China. Some areas have become known for certain types of jade. Many people think jade is only green, but really it can also be white, yellow, and black. Often there are different hues of a color. For instance white jade may have streaks of a cream color, and green jade might have a lighter streak imbedded in the jade. The value of jade depends on its sheen, uniformity, texture, and strength. Which one of these pieces do you like the best?"

Pei Ke looked for a few minutes and pointed to a jade amulet.

"You have an ability to recognize the finer qualities of jade. Would you like to wear it around your neck to see how it looks?"

"How much is it?"

"You should take the amulet that you have around your neck off first so you can try this one on."

Pei Ke's hand immediately went to his chest to make sure the amulet he was wearing was still there. With a sense of relief he turned to look at Liu who was deep in thought.

"Thank you," said Liu. "We are poor travelers and could not afford such an exquisite work of art. Thank you for your time and your words. They were very educational."

Bowing to the shopkeeper, Liu turned away and motioned for Pei Ke to follow. Both men wondered whether the request for Pei Ke to take off the amulet had just been a coincidence.

They were no more than thirty steps from the shopkeeper when Liu turned to look at him. He was talking to someone. The person seemed familiar to Liu, but he couldn't quite place him. Liu looked at Pei Ke and was going to say something, but changed his mind and said instead.

"Pei Ke while we are in Beijing I want you to see a shop I used to visit on a regular basis. We are very close to it."

They walked a couple of blocks. Liu looked at some of the signs, trying to remember the correct direction. As he turned to look at the shop in front of them, he realized he had arrived at his destination. They walked into the shop.

"Master, I am amazed to see all these books. I thought most books were written by hand and then copied by hand."

"Is this the first time you have seen printed books?"

"Well, no, Master," said Pei Ke. "I just did not give it much thought as to how the books were printed."

"Pei Ke, most people don't realize it, but China has a wealth of ancient inventions. We often take for granted the things we see and hear. Our culture has made major contributions to the development of mankind. The most notable and well known are paper, printing, gunpowder, and the compass."

"Master, what is a compass?"

"The compass is called Zhi Nan Zhen and literally means 'needle pointing south.' It is called this because it was believed that many of the important activities of China were in the south.

"It is a magnetized needle, balanced on a small pivot. The magnetized tip of the needle will align itself with the energy of the earth. It is used to help travelers and mariners travel in a continuous direction for extended periods of time.

"Traditionally, its creation was attributed to Huang Di, the Yellow Emperor. However, historical records also indicate that Ma Jun, who lived during the Three Kingdoms Period, helped to further develop the compass. To make it more confusing for you, there is some indication in the classic works that Shen Kuo of the Northern Song Dynasty wrote about a magnetized needle that was allowed to float on water to give directions to the travelers.

"Over the years the compass has been useful to our mariners. It has helped the ship captains travel to all parts of the world and to make discoveries that would never have been made without the compass. Many of the exotic things not native to China you see in Beijing are due to the sea captains having brought these items back from distant lands."

"Master, have you ever seen a compass?"

"Yes, when I was out at sea the captain of the ship had a compass. We were so far out we could not see land. It was only due to the compass that we knew which direction to travel."

"Couldn't you tell by the sun which way to go?"

"No, the sun travels across the sky. If we followed the sun we would be off by one hundred and eighty degrees."

"Why were you at sea?"

"I had an opportunity to be on a fishing vessel for a couple of days. The work is very hard and in some instances very dangerous."

"Master, now tell me about paper and printing."

"You first need to know how the Chinese characters were developed to get a full understanding about printing and paper. Our ancestors originally used pictorial representations. As an example, a round circle was used to indicate a 'mouth.' From the circle it developed into a square. As you know, if you put a line through the mouth you get the center or the middle. The meaning has changed and thus the pronunciation is different. Almost all Chinese characters can be broken down into parts that give the character meaning."

"Master, I remember my mother teaching me to read and write. She didn't go into a lot of detail on the derivation of the characters. My guess is she didn't know all the details about the historical development of each one of the characters."

"Since many of the characters have a historical development, you can understand and memorize the characters based on their individual components. It would not make sense to eliminate part of the character. It was one of the ancient emperors who decided that everyone needed to be able to understand his edicts so he standardized the writing of all characters. He insisted that throughout the land, everyone learn how to write each character in a certain way. My guess is it would have been impossible to require everyone to pronounce the characters the same, so he let the people pronounce them however they wanted as long as everyone in the land could read his edicts. Thus today we have one written language but many different dialects."

"Master, give me an example of the different dialects you have heard in all your travels."

Liu thought for a moment. There must be hundreds of dialects and he had only heard a few of them.

"Let me give you an example. The character for a person's hand is pronounced 'sew' in Beijing. In the south, around Hong Kong, it is pronounced 'sui.' In Fukien province, it is pronounced 'chui.' Another example is a person's eye. In Beijing, it is pronounced 'yen'. In Hong Kong, it is 'ngan.' In Fukien province it is 'bak.'

Liu went on to show Pei Ke the development of different characters and how their pictorial design gave a hint as to the meaning of the character.

"Master, now that you have explained the development of the characters and writing will you please tell me more about the development of paper."

"Did you know that before there was paper, the characters were written on bamboo strips hooked together? We read top to bottom so each line of words started at the top of the bamboo strip and continued downward. When the bottom of the strip was reached, the sentence resumed again at the top of the next strip to the left. This continued on until the end of the strips. One of the very old manuscripts I carry with me was written on bamboo strips."

"What does it say?"

Liu thought for a moment, hesitant to answer the question.

"The ancients experimented with different herbs and combinations of herbs. In many pieces of written folklore, mention is made of the various elixirs for longevity. I believe there is a basic formula that will prolong life and based on the person's constitution at birth, there are certain herbs to add or subtract from the basic formula.

"Since there are numerous herbal constitution patterns, there would be numerous herbal formulas. The old bamboo strips are a key to some of the information. I have some of the information and Uncle Wu has another piece, and Wei Ken De has another piece. When all the strips are together then the information is invaluable. Apart the strips are appropriate for only the person who has the strips. This was done purposely by me to make sure this information does not fall into the wrong hands."

"Master...."

"Enough for now. You can ask me some questions later on. For now I just want you to think about what has transpired. You should be reviewing in your mind what you have learned so far."

Liu's thoughts turned to his studies with his mother on calligraphy and painting. He remembered when his mother taught him how to make black ink. They had an ink stone, which was a flat ornate carved stone. At one end of the flat stone there was a reservoir with water. The ink itself was a solid piece of black pitch that was dipped into the water and then rubbed on the flat surface of the stone. As the ink stick was rubbed on the stone, the water would turn black. The darkness of the ink and the thickness of the ink were controlled by the amount of rubbing.

He often watched his mother as she showed him the correct way to make the ink. After hours of practice, he understood the concept and in fact rather enjoyed the process of making ink. On many occasions, when his mother or father were painting or writing calligraphy, he would stand next to the table and make the ink for them.

He remembered his mother telling him how to hold the brush. For generations the ink brush was held in a particular manner. The brush was always directly in front of the nose. The shoulders were relaxed. The elbow was off the table. The mouth was closed. The tongue touched the roof of the mouth. As the strokes were made, there was a special way of breathing so the breathing would not affect the movement of the brush. Liu felt that when he practiced calligraphy and painting, it was a way to be in touch with the Universal Energy. The more he practiced, the more he was able to relax into peacefulness. The peacefulness he experienced was similar to the peacefulness of the internal martial arts he had practiced later in life. He found it strange that many of the other boys his age did not sense the same thing he had sensed, but he had known at an early age that he was going to be different.

Liu and Pei Ke spent the whole day exploring various parts of the city. It brought back many memories for Liu. For Pei Ke it was an exciting opportunity to see a big city. He made many comparisons between what he saw in Beijing and what he knew from living in the countryside.

# CHAPTER FORTY-ONE

The next day they rose early as usual. After a quick cup of hot tea, they stepped out into the fresh early morning air. They walked several blocks. Liu seemed to know where he was going. There were others on the street going in the same direction, and Pei Ke assumed everyone was heading for the park.

He was right. After several turns they arrived at the entrance to the park. There were two stone columns, one on each side of the entrance. A sign across the top announced in bright red characters the name of the park. The first glimpse of morning light was on the distant horizon as they and others entered into the park.

Liu sensed a change in the Universal Energy as they passed the portal. He looked at Pei Ke. He could tell Pei Ke sensed it also, but it was only a cursory experience. Pei Ke was only mildly in tune with his body and senses.

"Master, have you ever been to this park before?"

"Yes, I came many years ago when I was training here in Beijing. I wanted you to see for yourself some of the better martial arts teachers. It is not always possible to go visit each one of them. Many of them I do not know, but it is always an education to see what others are doing.

"Many of these teachers rise early in the morning and come to this and other parks throughout Beijing to practice. Often they have some of their senior students join them."

"Master, how early do they get up? It is early in the morning and the park is already quite full."

"I can't answer for each one of them, but they are usually here between five and five-thirty in the morning. They usually will practice for about two hours and will be gone by seven-thirty. After practice they usually go out to breakfast with either some of the other teachers or with their senior students. The younger students are left to continue training or, if need be to go to work."

Liu and Pei Ke walked around the park. The morning chill and the stillness of the air invigorated them both. Liu had always liked the morning air. There was something clean about it, as though the Universal Energy had had an opportunity during the night to revitalize itself and prepare the world for the next day. He always noticed that early in the morning, people greeted each other on the street as they passed. Almost like the birds who call to each other first thing in the morning.

They passed many who were also walking around the park and Liu nodded in acknowledgement as they passed. Liu would stop occasionally and watch those practicing a certain style of martial arts. Pei Ke thought he was looking at the beauty of the constantly flowing movements, but in reality, he was analyzing the movements to see their simplicity.

Liu knew there were many expansive movements in Chinese martial arts. They looked beautiful to watch, but from his experience in real life situations it was the simple and direct movements that were the most effective. That was why he liked the three internal martial arts.

"Master, can I learn some of these martial arts? They are so beautiful to watch."

"There are hundreds of martial arts within China, and it is not possible for you to learn more than a couple of them. For many it takes a lifetime to understand the intricacies and implications of each. It is not possible to do justice to an art without years of training and dedicated practice. I am always leery of those who claim they have mastered numerous martial arts systems. Be happy with what you have and perfect the arts you already know. I realize sometimes it may be discouraging for you, but you need to understand you are no different than others who have learned these arts."

Pei Ke knew he shouldn't have asked the question. He really was happy with what he had and was just taken up with the beauty of the movements.

"Master, you're right. From what I already know, it is going to take me a lifetime to master just what you are willing to teach me. I'm grateful for you to have me as a student. I meant no disrespect with what I said; it was just the beauty of the movements that attracted me."

As they walked around the park, Pei Ke could see the park was becoming even more crowded. He realized some were doing martial arts while others were doing some version of Qi Gong and still others were doing stretching exercises.

As they passed a rather large boulder, Pei Ke saw an elderly man laying on the ground stretching. Pei Ke couldn't believe what he saw. The man had his legs stretched in opposite directions. His chin was placed close to his toes of one foot. The man had to be quite elderly, maybe in his late sixties to early seventies. Liu saw the same man.

"Master, how does he do that?"

"To be able to do that, one needs to practice all his life. This is his method of staying in good condition. Have you ever noticed that many animals, especially dogs and cats, stretch when they first wake up?"

"Yes, it is quite common for animals to do that. I just never thought of it as their way of strengthening their muscles."

Liu and Pei Ke nodded to the old man on the ground, and continued their walk. The park was meticulously cared for. Each section of the park had a different species of trees. A few vendors with their push carts provided hot soy bean drinks. One vendor had Yue Tiao and Shao Bing for sale.

The Yue Tiao was a foot long piece of dough that had been deep fried in oil. When the raw dough was placed in the hot oil, it quickly expanded so the cooked dough was hollow. It was placed on a piece of fried bread. Sometimes a fried egg was included. Pei Ke suspected there was no nutritional value to the Yue Tiao, but he had had it before and knew it was delicious. He was going to mention it to Liu, but thought better of the idea. Maybe they would eat later.

He was surprised not to see or smell his favorite smelly tofu. Maybe it was too much for the morning crowd.

They continued walking until Liu motioned for them to sit on a concrete bench. As they sat down, Pei Ke noticed a group of students who were practicing Pa Kua Chang. Immediately Pei Ke took an interest in what they were doing. They sat there for about ten minutes before Pei Ke asked.

"Master, I know they are practicing Pa Kua Chang by the characteristic movements of walking a circle and the palm changes. However, it doesn't look the same as what you've been teaching me."

Pei Ke was expecting an answer, but Liu just continued to sit and watch the students as they followed their teacher. It took all of Pei Ke's effort to keep quiet and not ask the question again. He would have to be patient.

Out of the corner of his eye, Pei Ke noticed Liu's hands resting on his thighs. This was not unusual except Liu's index finger was moving in a unique circular pattern. Pei Ke looked at the students who were practicing on the grass. Liu was tracing their movements with his finger. As they made a turn his finger would make a turn. Then he noticed Liu's head was slightly moving to the movement of his index finger. He'd never seen Liu do that before. He couldn't figure out if Liu was just following the movements to be in harmony with their flow or if he was trying to memorize the pattern. He couldn't imagine why Liu would need to memorize any more patterns.

When he could wait no longer, he opened his mouth to ask, but Liu cut him off.

"Just watch the students and pay particular attention to the teacher. If you have questions, you may ask me later. Observe what is happening."

Pei Ke watched the group practicing their Pa Kua Chang routines. He realized that most of the individual movements were similar to those he already knew. The difference was in the position of the hands and the stepping pattern. There were some movements he'd never seen, and of the movements he could recognize, the order of the movements was different from what he had learned.

He also noticed that the movements were more expansive than the ones he knew, almost to the point of being flowery. He was sure Liu was going to make a critical evaluation of the experience.

Ten minutes later, the group of students took a break and Liu, without any hint, stood and motioned for Pei Ke to follow him.

The park was huge. It had to be at least ten to fifteen acres in overall size. In the center of the park was a pavilion where some older men were sitting on benches and smoking. Pei Ke found it interesting that men came to the park to exercise but some also smoked. From what Liu had told him he knew smoking was detrimental to one's health. He remembered Liu mentioning that there were some very famous martial arts masters in China who had shortened their lives by smoking opium or drinking excessive amounts of plum wine.

As he scanned the park, he realized there were very few women there. Those who were in the park were older and not doing martial arts, but rather a form of stretching or Qi Gong. He surmised most of the women had to remain at home to watch over either their children or grandchildren.

A gust of cold air blew through the park, reminding them of the harshness of winter. It was not as cold here as it was in the mountains where they lived, but it was cold enough that he had to wear a coat. It was interesting to watch the martial artists in the park do their routines and see the puffs of air coming from their mouths as they exhaled.

They had walked around almost half the park when Liu again abruptly sat down. As Pei Ke sat down next to Liu, he understood why his master had stopped in that particular spot. In the distance, partially hidden behind some trees, there was a group of students practicing Hsing-Yi Chuan. They were dutifully following the lead of their instructor. Pei Ke could hear him calling off commands and watched the students execute these with military-like precision.

This time, they were far enough away from the group that Liu could speak without being overheard.

"Pei Ke."

"Yes, Master."

"Do you recognize what they are practicing?"

"Of course, Master. They are practicing Hsing-Yi Chuan."

"Do you know what movement within Hsing-Yi Chuan they are practicing?

"They are practicing Pi Chuan."

"I want you to watch it for a few minutes to see the essence of the way they execute the move of Pi Chuan."

Pei Ke watched intently. Liu had already taught him Pi Chuan. He had been practicing the movement, but it was different from what he now saw the group do. He studied the movement the students were doing. At first he couldn't quite put it into words why their Pi Chuan was different, but after a few minutes, he thought he knew the difference.

"What is the difference between what I have taught you and what you see these students doing?"

Pei Ke was about to reply when Liu continued.

"There are a number of differences. It doesn't mean that what I taught you is right or wrong, but these are stylistic differences and developmental differences that you should know and understand. By looking at the stepping pattern, the way they open the form, and the coordination between the hands and feet, one can differentiate if the basic style is from Hopei, Honan, or from some other background.

Liu went on to explain the differences between the various methods of doing Pi Chuan and how it related to the development in a particular area of China. Pei Ke found it interesting that Hsing-Yi Chuan, which originally came from Yue Fe hundreds of years earlier, had developed differently in different areas of China. He also found it interesting that some systems of Hsing- Yi Chuan had ten animal styles and others had twelve. After listening to the explanation from Liu, as to why they did it the way they did and Liu emphasizing that one method is not necessarily better than another, he was thankful he learned it the way he had.

For the next hour, they continued their walk around the park. They stopped occasionally when there was a place to sit. When it was appropriate, Liu would share with Pei Ke information about what they saw. Pei Ke had never seen such a divergent accumulation of different styles and systems in his whole life. He knew enough to identify which movements could be used in close quarters combat and which could not. He could tell when they were practicing warm-up exercises, strengthening exercises, forms, or drills.

"Pei Ke we need to be going. As you can see, the people are starting to leave. Many of them have to go to work and of course they don't want to be late."

"Master, is there anyone here you know?"

"It has been too long since I was last here to know or recognize anyone. Some of the very best teachers do not teach here. They prefer the privacy of their own homes. They stay away from drawing attention to themselves."

They walked around the last section of the park as more and more people were leaving. Pei Ke could see by their perspiration and the way they covered up against the cold wind that many had worked hard.

As they approached the exit to the park, Liu slowed and put his hand out to stop Pei Ke. Directly in front of them, not more than ten feet away, stood an old man with a long white beard and exceedingly long eyebrows. He was smiling with his hands on his hips.

"Liu, I heard you were back in Beijing and I knew I would find you here," said the old man. "So you have returned. How many years has it been since we last crossed arms?"

"It has been a few," said Liu. "Probably more than I can count. I see the gods have looked favorably on you. You seem to be in good health and have prospered well these many years I have been away."

"I have not done too badly. You are still the same. You will probably never change, even if a hundred years pass between us. The last time we saw each other was just before your departure. You never told anyone where you were going, though of course, there were rumors about where you went and what you were doing. There was even a rumor you had a wife hidden someplace to the west, but I knew you would never marry. So, where have you been all this time?"

"I decided it was in my best interest to seclude myself so I could practice and meditate. It was the peacefulness that kept me away all these years."

"I remember the last evening you were here; it was over at Teacher's house. You and I were pushing hands together. If I remember correctly, it was unanimously agreed by everyone that it was a draw."

"I do not remember," said Liu. "I said goodbye to Teacher and left."

"You never came back to see Teacher."

"We corresponded on numerous occasions. He sent me quite a few letters over the years," said Liu.

"I don't believe it," said the elderly man. "Teacher never mentioned it to any of us."

"I always let him know what I was doing and where I was living. When he passed away, his wife sent me a note and I responded to it. I felt it best not to return for the funeral given the circumstances of my departure.

"As you know," said Liu, my name appears on the official announcement of his death as one of his inner door students. I believe it is next to your name. Is that not correct?"

Pei Ke could see the man's demeanor change over the course of the conversation. Pei Ke sensed a lot of anger in the man's voice. He only sensed calm and peacefulness from Liu.

"What brings you back now?" said the other man.

As Pei Ke listened to the conversation he realized that there were many things about Liu and his past that were never mentioned to him. He wondered what else would be revealed about his teacher.

"The years have passed and I am sure many have forgotten the past or have let their hearts mellow over the years. In the twilight of my life, I would like to come back to visit with old friends and show my student the sights and sounds of this fair city. At one time, you and I were close friends. We trained together for many long hours. Maybe that could happen once again."

"How is your push hands ability?"

"We were always evenly matched," said Liu. "I am confident we have both progressed over the last decade or so. I expect you have had many students now since Teacher has passed away"

"Yes, I have had quite a few," said the man. "Many of Teacher's younger students came to me when he died. I don't teach here in the park. I only came because someone saw you yesterday on the street and recognized you from earlier years. I came to see for myself. Like Teacher, we keep our training to ourselves and away from the prying eyes of others. Did you ever share with others what you were taught?"

"Over the years I have had a few students; nothing like the numbers you have. You have done well for yourself."

"Is he any good?" said the old man pointing to Pei Ke.

"He is doing fine."

"He is the only one you have, right?" said the old man with a slight smirk on his face.

Liu never answered the question.

Pei Ke looked at the old man and then at Liu. He couldn't believe what he was seeing. Liu must have secrets Pei Ke had never suspected. This old man had quite a bit of animosity toward Liu, but Pei Ke didn't sense any from Liu had toward the old man. He was perfectly calm, even as the older man was getting more and more agitated.

Abruptly, the conversation stopped. Both men looked at each other silently. Pei Ke couldn't tell if they were sizing each other up or choosing their next words carefully.

After what seemed an eternity, Liu turned slightly to Pei Ke and motioned for him to follow. He never took his eyes off the man. Pei Ke looked at Liu and then at the older man in front of him. Pei Ke could tell Liu didn't trust the man. His master had his head turned in such a way that he could watch the old man as they departed.

"Master, who...."

"Later."

Pei Ke had hundreds of questions to ask, but it was obvious Liu didn't want to talk. Pei Ke tried to remember if he'd ever seen any friction between Liu and anyone else. The only thing Pei Ke could think of was the attack by the Chen family, and Liu had more or less defeated that group.

It was unfortunate that Chen's son had gotten away. Pei Ke wondered what else was in Liu's background. He almost wished there would have been a contest between Liu and the other man. Maybe it will still happen while they are in Beijing.

They were to go back to the park one more time. Pei Ke didn't realize it at the time but his own martial arts skills would be tested.

# CHAPTER FORTY-TWO

The street they walked down was no different than many of the streets that Pei Ke had seen throughout their travels. It had its accumulation of trash and various hand written notices on the walls with messages of everything one could think about. The crowd of early morning shoppers was starting to thin out a little.

"Master, I have never been in such a big city before. There is everything here one could ever want."

"There are many things here; almost too many things. It is easy to become distracted and lose track of why one has come in the first place. We are here to meet with some of my old friends and acquaintances and visit places you have never seen before. This may be your only visit to Beijing."

"Master, what is this area we are in now? It has an unusual look and feel to it."

"This is one of the oldest areas of Beijing. We are going to walk through it so you can see its uniqueness."

They walked down numerous streets. They stopped walking and were looking at the beautiful apples at a fruit stand when Liu looked up to see a man staring intently at him. Liu didn't know why he looked up. Maybe it was his inner sense always warning him of impending danger. Whatever it was, Liu immediately positioned himself between Pei Ke and the man watching him.

"Master, these apples look delicious. Let's get one for each of us."

Liu looked at the two apples Pei Ke held in his hand.

"How are you going to pay for them? They are not free."

Pei Ke disliked being poor. It was like a curse inflicted on the many by the few. Maybe he should have made a different decision at the temple before he started after Liu. He put the two apples back on the pile and looked down at the ground. Liu turned to look at the man who'd been staring at him, but the man was gone. Liu quickly scanned the area. The first man was gone, but there was another staring at him.

"Pei Ke, forget the apples. Let's leave."

"There are other stalls with many items. I know we cannot buy them, but it's always nice to see what is available. Let's look at a couple more vendors."

"Pei Ke, we should go now!"

Pei Ke suddenly sensed Liu's urgency.

"Master, what's wrong?"

"I don't know yet, but the situation may be developing unfavorably for us. There was a man watching us intently for some time. He has been replaced by another. I want to avoid any trouble."

Liu quickly led them away in the direction they had come. They had gone no more than thirty feet when Liu saw both men approaching. At first, they were walking slowly, but they suddenly picked up the pace as they drew near. Liu knew something was going to happen, but he couldn't tell yet where the attack was going to come from.

Pei Ke wondered if his master would bring out the knife hidden up his sleeve or wait for the attack and then bring it out. He had no more than thought of it when one of the men drew his own knife from his pocket. Pei Ke and Liu saw it at the same time.

The two men were now only six feet away. They were separated and one stabbed at Liu's stomach. The other rushed toward Pei Ke.

Liu mentally calculated the distance of the knife to his body and stepped immediately to his left. He slightly raised his right hand just before the knife made contact and sliced downward with the outside of his right hand against the outside of the right hand of the assailant, deflecting the knife to the right. As the knife moved away, Liu stepped in and twisted the opponent's wrist in a painful Chin Na move designed to twist the knife towards the assailant himself. The man dropped the knife and twisted away. Immediately, Liu knew his opponent was familiar with martial arts. Very few people knew how to get out of that Chin Na move. The man immediately changed the angle of the Chin Na attack to his advantage and Liu was now on the defensive.

The second man grabbed Pei Ke's right arm and started to pull him away. Pei Ke struggled to get out of the forceful grip, fear quickly overcoming him. The more he struggled the more he realized he was not going to win. The man was just too strong for him. Deep in the recesses of his mind he remembered that Liu had told him to relax in these types of situations. But how could he relax when he was certain he was going to get hurt?

Pei Ke forced himself to relax. The man interpreted it as weakness and started to twist Pei Ke's arm. Pei Ke lowered his body just enough so his elbow was directly below his wrist. This twisted the man's arm just enough to put pressure against the thumb. Pei Ke could feel the grip relaxing as he started to twist out of the grab.

Pei Ke realized he needed to do something quickly and instinctively applied one of the Chin Na moves Liu had taught him. He didn't know how much force to use so he used as much as he could apply. He heard the man yell and felt the joint of the man's wrist turn downward as he broke the man's wrist in one single downward motion.

The man who'd attacked Liu fared even worse. His arm was broken and his shoulder was dislocated. Liu surveyed the scene. Pei Ke was startled and didn't know what to do next. A crowd was starting to assemble and Liu didn't want to be the center of attention.

"Let's go," said Liu. He motioned for Pei Ke to follow and they quickly left their attackers to the increasing crowd. They both looked back when they were twenty feet away.

"Are you all right?" asked Liu.

"Yes," said Pei Ke. "It happened so fast I didn't have time to think. Why did they attack us?"

"I don't know, but we are not going to stay around and find out. I don't know the mood of the crowd."

Liu had not had time to watch what Pei Ke had done but he was pleased to see the results. Pei Ke was finally becoming a martial artist.

# CHAPTER FORTY-THREE

The next morning they had breakfast at a little shop close to where they were staying. It was a family business with not more than ten tables and it appeared that each family member was assigned something to do. The husband cooked and the wife collected money. The children cleaned the dishes, swept the floor, and poured the tea. It was an efficient operation. As they waited in line, Pei Ke could smell the cooking oil used in preparing the different foods.

They waited in line for the hot, sweetened soy bean drink, Yue Tao, and onion cake. Onion cake was one of Pei Ke's favorite morning staples. His mother had cooked it for him. He marveled at the many different ways restaurants cooked it. Many prepared the onion cake thick, but he preferred it thin with a large helping of chives or green onions blended inside the dough. Some cooks only fried it lightly. He liked his fried on a hot skillet and cooked crispy. This restaurant cooked it just the way his mother cooked it.

They found an empty table in the back corner. Liu sat with his back to the wall, giving him an unobstructed view of who came and went.

"Pei Ke, after we finish eating, we are going to visit one of my teacher's graves. I would like to pay respect to him while we are in Beijing."

"Master, while we are eating is it all right for me to ask you some questions about acupuncture?"

"What questions do you have?"

"Am I correct in thinking that some acupuncture points are more important than others?"

"Important is one way to put it. I would say that we use certain acupuncture points more often than others because they have a broader range of therapeutic effects. In addition, these points are used more frequently in combination with other points.

"Do you remember me telling you about Ma Dan Yang a few months ago? He identified ten acupuncture points he felt were vital for the acupuncturist to know. Later generations added two more points. We know these points now as the Twelve Ma Dan Yang Points. They are so important that during the course of a day's practice the doctor will have used these points numerous times.

"Let me give you an example. The acupuncture point Tsu San Li is one of the twelve Ma Dan Yang points. It is on the Stomach Meridian and is located just below the knee on the outside of the leg. There are a couple of different ways to locate this point, which I will show you later. It is only a matter of preference and how you were trained to locate it.

"The point refers to ancient China when many individuals had to walk long distances. When their legs and feet became tired and sore, they would use this point to stimulate the energy so they could walk farther. Of course, the name literally means 'foot three miles,' but we interpret it to mean the use of the point relieves the stress in the legs and feet.

"As an interesting note, this point is located three human inches below the knee cap. Do you remember what a human inch is and how to measure it?"

"Yes, Master. The human inch is not the measure from the measuring stick. Rather it is the standard measuring criteria used to measure distances on the human body so we can locate the same acupuncture point whether it is on an infant or on an adult."

"Good.

"Since this is one of the main points on the Stomach Meridian, it is useful in treating any type of stomach problem, including digestive problems, vomiting, indigestion, diarrhea, constipation, abdominal discomfort, and weight problems.

"Because the pathway of the meridian is in close proximity to the lateral side of the knee, the point is quite often used to treat knee problems including sprains, strains, arthritis, inflammation, and bruises.

"The pathway of the Stomach Meridian goes to the chest and across the breast so it can be used to treat women's breast problems such as mastitis, lack of lactation, and breast pain. I have even used it to treat women who have had severe injuries to their breasts where part of the breast tissue had been cut away. They were in pain for years and this point relieved their discomfort. Of course I used other points in conjunction with this point to treat this problem. Can you imagine having this pain for many years? It is a shame women have to suffer when it can be treated.

"Now Pei Ke, do you remember where on the Stomach Meridian it is located?"

"Yes, Master, I remember." Pei Ke pointed to the area on his body that corresponded to the Stomach Meridian.

"Good. You remembered. This point on the leg has also been used to treat dizziness, insomnia, headaches, and various types of mental disorders.

"In theory any acupuncture point along a meridian should be able to help with the flow of energy. Remember, all we are doing when we insert the needle is balancing the flow of energy so the body can return to a normal condition for that particular body. I believe this to be true, but the ancients found certain points like Tsu San Li and others, which have a better effect on the body and the meridian.

"As such, this is one of those points on the Stomach Meridian that can treat any problem lying along its pathway. This is why it is important to memorize the pathway of each meridian. There are some meridians that are in close proximity to another and it would be better to get the correct meridian when you are doing a treatment.

"There are a number of therapeutic actions possible with Tsu San Li point. Since it is on the Stomach Meridian, it can harmonize the stomach, especially if there is a feeling of heat in the stomach area. Since it is a Yang Meridian, it helps the Yin coupled Meridian, which is the Spleen Meridian, and we can use this point in conjunction with the Spleen Meridian to treat diarrhea.

"This is such a wonderful point and I find it useful in just about everything dealing with enhancing Qi in the body.

"I remember one of my teachers telling me this point is one of the major points to help with good health and longevity. Routine moxibustion on this point will go a long way in helping to fight off the aging process. It is especially good for older individuals experiencing a decrease in overall vitality. Of course, like everything else, you should not overdue it, but you need to be consistent with weekly treatments. You probably won't see any true benefits until you have done it for awhile.

"The famous acupuncturist Gao Wu considered the Tsu San Li point to be so important, he classified it as one of the four major acupuncture points on the body. These four points treat a wide range of health care issues. After his death, later acupuncturists added two more points. The original four points and the two that were added have come to be known as the Six Command Points."

"Master, what are the Six Command Points?"

"They are Lie Que on the Lung Meridian, He Gu on the Large Intestine Meridian, Tsu San Li on the Stomach Meridian, Wei Zhong on the Bladder Meridian, Nei Guan on the Pericardium Meridian, and Ren Zhong on the Governing Vessel Meridian. Do you think you can remember these six acupuncture points? I realize you do not know how to locate them all, but for now just remember them."

"Yes, Master. I will remember."

"Pei Ke, you have enough information on the Tsu San Li acupuncture point. Do you have any specific questions about the therapeutic benefits or advantages of using this point?"

"No, Master, but I would like it if you could share information on another one of the Six Command Points. I think I can remember more. Which one of the six points would be most appropriate for me to know?"

"I think you should know Nei Guan. It is known as the 'Inner Pass' point and is on the Pericardium Meridian. It is located on the inside of arm just above the wrist crease. It is a Yin Meridian and its opposite Yang Meridian is the Triple Warmer Meridian, which is on the outside of the arm and is referred to as the 'Outer Pass.' So there is the Inner Pass and the Outer Pass. This is one way for you to remember these two points."

"Master can you show me how to locate this point?"

Liu took Pei Ke's left arm and turned it over so the inside of the arm was facing up. He took Pei Ke's fingers and showed him exactly how to locate the point.

"Master, if Nei Guan is on the inside and Wei Guan is on the outside and one point is above the other, these two points are in very close proximity to each other. Am I correct?"

"Yes, you are correct. In fact, there are many instances where it is appropriate to use one needle to stimulate both points. The technique is a little too advanced for you now. Just remember how to locate the points."

"Wouldn't that cause discomfort to the patient?"

"There would be no discomfort to the patient if done properly. It isn't any different than inserting the needle anywhere else on the body, but as I said, you shouldn't worry about that now.

"Nei Guan is a very useful point for any type of heart problem, like palpitations and heart pain. It is very effective in treating nausea and vomiting. I use this point to treat women when they have morning sickness. In conjunction with Gong Sun, it can be used to treat any type of chest or intercostal pain. Since the Pericardium Meridian transverses the chest, it can be used to treat a wide range of lung problems, including cough and asthma. Also, we could treat your mother's insomnia with it, along with other points. Of course, since this point lies on the Pericardium Meridian and the Pericardium Meridian goes from the chest area down the arm to the hand, this point is effective in treating shoulder, elbow, and wrist problems.

"Do you remember a few months ago when I spoke of Connecting Points?"

"Yes, Master."

"Nei Guan is the Connecting Point on the Pericardium Meridian. It is at this point that the energy of the Pericardium Meridian passes on to its coupled meridian, the Triple Warmer Meridian.

"Is that too confusing for you?"

"No, actually, it's not confusing at all. The more I learn, the easier it is for me to have a concept of acupuncture and how it works on the body. The only problem I have is trying to remember everything."

"We all have the same problem. It is important to have significant amounts of clinical experience so you can remember the points and what they represent before you are ever on your own as a doctor. There are some practitioners who think they can master this art by just reading the ancient texts or listening to the doctor. There is no substitute for the experience a seasoned practitioner has acquired.

"Pei Ke, this is enough for you to remember for now. I want to finish my meal."

For a time, they both ate in silence. Liu was thinking of his teachers, and Pei Ke was thinking alternately of what Liu had taught him and of the good restaurants he had visited in the short time he had been in Beijing. He wondered how many more days they would stay.

"Pei Ke, you must be finished by now. I know the food is good, but too much of a good thing is bad for you. It is like the Universal Tao. When the Yin aspect of the Tao becomes too excessive, it changes into its counterpart, the Yang aspect of the energy. If you consistently eat too much, the energy of your body is going to change and it may not be for the better. Enjoy your food, but it is always best to eat slowly and eat only enough to sustain you. Anything more is unhealthy."

When they were finished eating, Liu rose.

"Be sure and pay the owner for this nice meal," he said. "Use those coins jingling in your pocket."

Pei Ke was going to say something but thought better of it.

After leaving the restaurant they went to a cemetery on the outskirts of Beijing for Liu to pay respect to two of his acupuncture teachers and one of his martial arts teachers.

# CHAPTER FORTY-FOUR

Pei Ke, today we are going to a clinic in the center of Beijing. Years ago, I spent a considerable amount of time there helping the doctors when they were short of trained practitioners. There has always been an open invitation for me to return."

Liu and Pei Ke walked along one of the main thoroughfares toward the city center. Pei Ke had never seen so many people on a street at one time. Everyone was in a hurry. It seemed like orderly chaos. In this area of the city the buildings were larger and taller than he had ever seen before. Looking down the narrow alleys, he could see clothes hanging on ropes stretched across the alley from one building to another. The smells and sights were enough to keep him in constant amazement. They walked for about forty-five minutes until they came to large building in the middle of the block. The sign indicated it was a women's and children's hospital. Liu looked around then walked up the three steps to the entrance.

As he entered, a wave of thoughts flooded through his brain. He recalled the many days and nights he'd spent here treating patients. He thought of the many successes he had and the occasional failure. Knowing what he knew now, those who had not benefited from his treatments then would certainly benefit now. Experience was a primary factor in his art and he hoped Pei Ke would realize what needed to be done to be a good practitioner.

262 • Richard A. Peck

The entrance way had not changed in the years since he had last been there. Over to the right, an area for jackets was almost full to capacity, just as it was many years previous. As he walked toward the registration desk, he passed a large group of women with toddlers of all ages. There were a couple of men fidgeting nervously, who were most likely with their wives.

Liu and Pei Ke approached the registration desk and queued up behind about twenty others. Liu looked at the women in line and some who were sitting in the waiting area. From their faces and the way they carried themselves, he could tell there was a lot of suffering. This was going to be an educational experience for Pei Ke.

"May I help you?" asked the woman behind the desk when they finally made their way up to the reception desk. Liu could tell from the tone of her voice that she was already stressed from the patient load, though it was still only morning. She looked up and there was instantaneous recognition. She had changed only a little over the years and was as beautiful as ever. Memories flooded his mind as he looked at Ming Hong for the first time in over a decade. He didn't know if she recognized him.

"Is Dr. Lang here?" asked Liu.

Ming Hong looked at him for the longest time before answering and Liu could see the recognition in her eyes and her faint smile. Liu felt the searching eyes as she looked deep into his. Not quite sure what to say after so long and clearly not sure if he recognized her, she hesitantly spoke.

"Dr. Lang is no longer here. He passed away a couple of years ago. Is there something I can do for you?"

"Many years ago I practiced acupuncture here. Who is in charge now?"

"What is your name?" asked the woman.

"Liu Bin."

She looked at him for a long time, her smile growing more confident. Slowly she rose and bowed to him.

"Master Liu, you do not remember me, but when you were here, you saved my life. A few months after you treated me, you departed under somewhat hurried and strange circumstances. I was so impressed with your healing ability and the work you did in the hospital I came to work here in the clinic. I always wondered where you went. I wondered when you would return. It is nice to see you back."

"I do remember you," said Liu. "We had tea together more than once." He smiled and they stared at each other for a few moments, each one of them bringing forth their individual memories.

"Master Liu, I have a son."

"You and your husband must be very proud. How many children do you have?"

"Only one. You must come and meet him. I have told him so much about you. His name is Ming Lo."

"I would like to meet him," said Liu. "How old is he?"

"Ten."

Liu and Ming Hong looked at each other for a few moments before she spoke.

"A few years after you left, Dr. Lang passed away. Dr. Hu, his assistant, took over for him and is still here. Do you remember him?"

As Pei Ke listened to the conversation, he watched the woman. He wasn't sure, but he thought he caught a widening of her eyes as she spoke. She was truly happy to see Liu. He looked at Liu and then back at the woman. He didn't know what it meant, but maybe there was more than what was being spoken. He quickly put it out of his mind.

"Yes, I remember him," said Liu. "Is he in today?"

"Yes, he is in, but he is making rounds with the other doctors. Follow me and you can wait in his office. I don't think he will mind."

Liu and Pei Ke followed Ming Hong to Dr. Hu's office. As they entered, the woman excused herself to look for the doctor. Liu watched her go. After a few moments he turned to Pei Ke.

"Pei Ke, I have been in this office many times. Actually, more times than I can remember. Some of the paintings on the wall are different and there are more books than before, but this office has not changed in many years. Dr. Lang, Dr. Hu, and I shared many conversations in this office over tea."

"Master, the woman you were talking to. Is she a friend?"

Liu looked at Pei Ke piercingly for a moment before he answered.

"It is as she said. She was a patient here, and I treated her."

Pei Ke was certain there was more to the story than that and it comforted him somehow. Maybe his master was human after all.

It was not long before Dr. Hu entered.

"Liu Bin," said Dr. Hu. "It's so good to see you again. I couldn't believe my ears when Ming Hong told me you were in my office waiting."

Liu introduced Dr. Hu to Pei Ke.

"So you are studying from Liu?"

"Yes, doctor," said Pei Ke.

"You are indeed fortunate. We all learned a lot about Traditional Chinese Medicine when Liu was working in the hospital, and we also knew that while he worked here, he was teaching us. This hospital is well known because of your teacher's efforts."

Hu turned to look at Liu.

"I see you have spoken with Ming Hong."

"Yes, it has been a long time since I have been here. She indicated she has a son now, and she wants me to meet him. Time seems to move so fast for all of us. Who did she marry?"

"Liu, she is not married," said Hu.

Liu and Hu stared at each other, neither saying a word. Finally, Hu said. "I believe you treated her when she was a patient at the clinic."

"Yes, I did."

"She needed a job, and we decided to let her work here. She has been with us ever since you departed. Every once in a while, your name would be mentioned by a patient who you had seen. You had quite a following while you were here. Many have asked where you went, but nobody knew for sure. We made some inquiries, but nobody seemed to know anything about your disappearance."

Liu did not answer. They just looked at each other.

"Liu, what brings you to Beijing? You departed rather mysteriously. There were many rumors, but I did not give any credence to them. You had your reasons, and knowing you were always an honorable person, I mentally wished you well, whatever you did and wherever you went."

"I have brought Pei Ke so he can visit some new places and meet some of my friends here. We have only been here a short time, but I wanted Pei Ke to see the hospital and, with your permission, spend some time in the hospital as an observer."

"You are both welcome. I assume you are going to make rounds with us. You can't possibly refuse me."

"Yes," said Liu. "I will join you and your staff and help out as much as possible."

———————

Later that day Liu and Pei Ke were making rounds with one of the resident doctors.

"Master," said the doctor. "This patient has come to us because she is experiencing repeated instances of morning sickness. She is two months pregnant. She started having morning sickness immediately after becoming pregnant."

Liu turned to the woman and asked.

"When did the morning sickness start?"

"Actually, I started having nausea and then I missed my period. I then suspected I was pregnant. So it has been maybe a month now since it started."

"I would like to go over the symptoms more specifically with you. I want you to tell me everything in detail."

"I feel very nauseous, especially in the morning. I often vomit after I eat, so it is difficult to keep food and liquid in my stomach. I do find it is much easier and I am less nauseous and vomit less if I just eat a few mouthfuls and wait, instead of eating a full meal."

"How does your chest feel?"

"It feels full, distended, and heavy."

"Are you alert or tired?"

"I have to stay alert because of my other children, but often feel tired and lazy. I force myself to do things. This pregnancy is different than my other two. With the other two, I had lots of energy, but this time I'm tired. Do you know what's wrong with me? Is my baby going to be all right?"

"Yes, your baby is going to be fine. This is a common thing, but there are several possible causes. Are you experiencing any other symptoms?"

"No."

"Do you feel angry or depressed?"

"No, I feel quite happy about the pregnancy. I hope it's going to be a boy. We have two girls, and we want a boy."

"Do you feel dizzy from the nausea?"

"No."

"When you vomit, does it taste really sour to you?"

"It doesn't taste pleasant, but I can't say it's really sour."

"Do you belch frequently, especially after eating?"

"I do belch, but not frequently."

"Are you experiencing any other symptoms that are different from when you were not pregnant?"

"No."

"Do you feel hot or cold?"

"Neither."

"Is there anything unique in the color, smell, or quantity of your urination?"

"No."

"Do you have any abdominal pain or contractions?"

"No."

"Other than being pregnant, do you feel bloated?"

"No."

"Do you have any breast tenderness or soreness?"

"Yes, I forgot to tell you that my breasts are tender, and they feel fuller, but this happened the last two times I was pregnant. I assumed it's a normal process."

"Yes, it is normal for your breasts to get larger as your body prepares itself for nursing your baby. I would only be concerned if the swelling or tenderness was excessive.

"I need to take your pulses to see if there is an imbalance in your energy."

"Do you need for me to lie down?"

"No, but I would like for you to stay seated and put your wrist on this small pillow. It will help me to take your pulses."

Liu adjusted the wrist pillow on the table so that her hand would be more comfortable. Before taking the pulses, Liu looked at the patient's skin, hair, and overall appearance. He did not detect any unusual conditions or smells. He felt the pulses on both the right and left sides, taking time to differentiate the quality of each pulse.

"Well, you are definitely pregnant."

"You can tell by taking my pulse?"

"Yes, in Traditional Chinese Medicine there is usually a distinct pulse combination for pregnancy—and you have it."

"Is it going to be a boy?"

Liu thought for a minute as he read the pulse. He knew what she wanted to hear, but felt it better for her to experience the beautiful feeling of the pregnancy.

"I am not certain if it is going to be a boy or girl. Does it matter to you?"

"Of course not, but it would be nice to have a boy. A boy will be able to take care of my husband and me in our old age."

"Would you please stick out your tongue?"

Liu noticed her tongue was pale with a white coating. If her tongue had been red, and the coating had been yellow, then he would have asked her some more questions.

"Pei Ke, come and look at her tongue. Remember what this looks like for future reference. Also feel her pulses so you can identify what a pregnant woman's pulse feels like."

Pei Ke did as he was told, first looking at the tongue, than feeling the pulses. He noted the quickness of the pulses and compared it mentally to other pulses he had felt.

"Based on the answers to my questions," Liu said when he was done, "the way you look, and your tongue and pulses, I feel you have an imbalance in your spleen and stomach energy."

"Is it serious?"

"No, it is typical and can be solved with acupuncture."

"What causes it?"

"From the point of view of Traditional Chinese Medicine, morning sickness is attributed to a combination of stomach Qi deficiency and a stoppage of the monthly period. When your body realizes there is a baby on the way, your energy patterns are disrupted. Sometimes this sudden change is too much for the woman's body, and other energy patterns become deficient. Don't worry, acupuncture can help this problem. You will need a few visits and then hopefully you will feel better and have a normal, happy pregnancy."

He turned to the other doctor and said, "Do you know how to handle this situation?"

"Yes, Master. We can use an acupuncture point on the Pericardium Meridian and an acupuncture point on the Spleen Meridian."

"Yes, and use the main stomach point on the leg to tonify the stomach and spleen energy. I would avoid the use of any abdominal points and any of the other contraindicated points during pregnancy. Do not use too much stimulation as we don't want the Qi to move too fast."

He turned to Pei Ke.

"Pei Ke, do you have any questions you want to ask?"

"Master, do all women who have morning sickness have the same pulses?"

"No two women are going to be exactly alike. This is true of all healthcare issues. However, since there is a close enough similarity between one woman and another, you can have a good deal of confidence if you feel these pulses again that you will know the woman is pregnant and has morning sickness.

"As I have mentioned to you before, it is a combination of many factors leading us to our differential diagnosis, however; in some cases certain factors weigh more heavily on our decision than others and you will learn to recognize these."

"Could there possibly be another reason she is experiencing morning sickness?"

"Yes, if she were to tell me a different set of symptoms then she would have a different underlying problem. For the patient it is the same, but for us doctors it is a different cause, requiring a different treatment pattern."

"Master, instead of acupuncture, would acupressure help with this problem?"

"Acupressure would give some temporary relief, but I don't think it would solve the underlying energy problem."

"Master, how soon will she see some relief from the morning sickness?"

"She should see some relief on this first treatment. I have seen instances where immediate relief is experienced as soon as the needles are inserted into the acupuncture points.

"Of course every woman is different, but from my experience she will need three to four visits in close succession for this to be completely successful."

"On the next visit would you expect the tongue and pulses to be the same?"

"Since she is pregnant, she will have the pulse of a woman who is pregnant, but she would have less of a pulse of someone who has morning sickness. It is important to differentiate the pregnant part of the pulses and the morning sickness part of the pulses. This is where experience is important.

"For this reason, there should be a close relationship between the doctor and the patient so the doctor can see the changes taking place in the diagnostic process. If this woman were to see a different doctor each time she came in, the doctor would not have the benefit of seeing the progress being made. Of course, the doctor can make a spot decision based on what he finds at the moment, but cannot make a decision based on progress, since he has no reference as to the starting point of the health care issue.

"This is why there needs to be a continuous, close relationship between doctor and patient. Without the continuity, the doctor will not be able to see the overall progress of the disease pattern and the healing process. Many times a close relationship with one doctor will allow the doctor to advise the patient on a developing pattern leading to potential future health care issues.

"Master, based on what you have seen in your differential diagnostic process, what other health care issues is this woman going to experience during her pregnancy?"

"I don't foresee any other problems developing, but it doesn't mean there won't be other problems during the nine-month gestation process."

"What could cause her to have problems?"

"Remember when you asked me what causes illness?"

"Yes, Master."

"Give me an answer. What causes illness?"

"All health care issues can be attributed to an imbalance of the energy in our bodies. Prevent or correct the imbalance and the body will be healthy and capable of healing itself."

"Good."

Pei Ke could see the woman was listening very intently to the conversation between him and his teacher.

"What do you suspect caused an imbalance in this woman's body?"

"I can't be sure," said Liu. "However, this problem can be due to irregular meals and diet. It can also be due to stressful life situations. She has two other children she needs to take care of in addition to a house and a husband. I suspect she has her hands full trying to manage everything and doesn't get regular meals and…."

"You are right," said the woman. "My husband works so hard to support the family, but it is not enough and I have to help out as much as I can and still take care of the children. I don't get regular meals and I always feel stressed over our life situation. I don't want to make it sound like I am complaining because I am not. It's just the reality of the situation."

"You will be fine," said Liu to the woman. "Try and reduce your stress and eat meals on a more regular basis."

Liu treated the woman. Later the three of them visited with other patients. At each patient, Liu and the doctor would discuss the patient's history and the symptoms of the health care issue. Liu would give his opinion and the doctor usually agreed as to the diagnosis and treatment pattern. They continued visiting patients for most of the day.

# CHAPTER FORTY-FIVE

The next day, Liu and Pei Ke arrived at the hospital early to start morning rounds. Liu decided to accompany the same doctor with whom he saw patients the previous day.

The doctor stopped at the bedside of a woman who had just arrived at the clinic. She looked distraught and held her infant close to her bosom.

"I see you have just arrived at the clinic," said the doctor. "What can we do for you?"

"My baby is two-weeks old, and I have very little breast milk to feed the baby. The midwife said my milk would come in shortly, but it has not come and I want to nurse my baby."

"Your baby is two-weeks old?"

"Yes."

"What have you been feeding your baby?"

"Water and soy bean milk, but I don't think it's enough."

"Master Liu would you like to consult with this woman while I see to some of the other patients?"

"Yes, of course."

Pei Ke watched as Liu introduced himself and Pei Ke to the young woman. It was obvious she was worried and a little apprehensive about what was going to happen to her and her child.

"Why did you come to this clinic?"

"I was told the doctors here see primarily woman and children."

"Yes, it is true."

"Are you one of the doctors here?"

"I am a consultant here in this clinic. I was here many years ago and have returned briefly to help out. I have seen many instances of the problem you are experiencing."

Pei Ke could see the instant relief on the patient's face. She looked down at her baby and then at Liu and smiled.

"Will you help me?"

"Of course, but I need to ask you some questions."

"That's fine."

"Did you have a normal pregnancy?"

"Yes. I was uncomfortable towards the end, but everything seemed normal to me."

"While you were pregnant, what did you eat?"

"We don't have a lot of money and sometimes we didn't have enough to eat."

"It is important to have a well-balanced diet, including plenty of soup made from bones. Fish is good for you and your baby. Is this your first child?"

"Yes but I had a miscarriage three years ago."

"How was the delivery?"

"It was very difficult. I was weak before the contractions started, and I had to push and bear down so hard. I could see the midwife was worried during the delivery. I was in labor for over twenty-four hours, and it was so painful. But it is such a joy to have a child. The midwife said there was more blood loss than normal. Does that make a difference?"

"It could," said Liu.

"How do you feel now?"

"Weak and tired. I'm not really hungry, but I know I need to eat for my baby."

"Yes, you need to eat and also you need to drink sufficient liquids to produce enough milk. If you don't drink enough then your body is going to be even weaker than it is now.

"Do your breasts feel full and distended? Are they painful?"

"They are not painful, but they do feel and look larger than they were before I was pregnant."

"Do they feel hot or warmer than usual?"

"No. Why?"

"If your breasts were hard and warm, it would be an indication you have an infection. An infection could also cause a lack of breast milk, but needs to be treated differently than a lack of breast milk without an infection. Do you have any milk at all?"

"Yes, there is a little but not enough. My baby always seems hungry. When I squeeze my breasts, I would expect milk to come out."

"Do you have any other health issues other than lack of milk?

"I am tired."

"Do you feel depressed or angry?"

"No, I'm quite happy to have this baby. We have tried for so many years. Even though she's a girl, she is a blessing to us. It is a sense of relief to have this child. My mother-in-law has been asking me over and over when we were going to start a family. Now I can have some peace with her."

"Where does your mother-in-law live?"

"My husband's parents live in the country many miles from here."

"Where are you staying now?"

"We were staying with friends during my pregnancy. Like us, they are very poor, but we are all happy, at least as happy as we can be under the circumstances. We need to stay here in Beijing because this is where my husband works. Neither of us wants to go back to the countryside."

"Where do your parents live?"

"They live in the same rural area as my husband's parents. The matchmaker set us up from birth. I did not meet him until I was fifteen. We were married shortly after and have been trying to have children ever since."

"How has your heart felt since the birth of your baby?"

She gave Liu a strange look.

"It's interesting you ask that question. Not always, but often, my heart beats so strongly that I've noticed it. Is there something wrong with my heart?"

"I don't believe so. It is just one more symptom to isolate the exact cause of your problem. Do you feel pain in your chest or abdomen?"

"No, but I'm still sore from the delivery. Does the soreness mean I will not be able to have more children?"

"No, the soreness just means you are healing from the delivery. It takes a while for a woman to recover after child birth. You will be fine, and should be able to have more children."

Pei Ke could see the happiness on the mother's face. She was worried, but seemed content. Pei Ke sensed she led a very simple, uncomplicated life without the demands one feels when living in a large city. In some aspects, he was like her.

"I need to feel your pulses and look at your tongue. Is that ok?"

"Why do you need to do that?"

"I have not finished diagnosing the problem you are having."

Liu picked up a chair and brought it over to the bed and sat down in the chair. He felt her pulses.

"Pei Ke, feel her pulses. Pay attention to the weak and thready pulses. They are an indication of a Qi and blood deficiency originating from the depletion of Qi during childbirth, and the excessive loss of blood during delivery."

Pei Ke felt the pulses and made a mental note of what he felt. He was sure he would be seeing this type of pulse again.

"Please stick out your tongue for me," said Liu.

Liu and Pei Ke both examined the tongue for its color, coating, shape, and any unusual markings. It was pale with little or no coating, indicating a deficiency. Liu pointed this out to Pei Ke, who made a mental note of the combination of the pulses and the tongue.

Liu looked at the mother and child and said. "From what you have told me and the signs and symptoms of your problem, you have a basic Qi and blood deficiency. It is not serious, but you must change your diet for the health of your baby and yourself. You need to drink more fluids, preferably soup, and eat plenty of vegetables and fish. Will you do this?"

"Yes, it is possible. Just this morning my husband told me he was getting a second job. We will have more money, and we can afford better food. But can you help me now with my problem? I really want to nurse my baby. Isn't she beautiful?"

"Yes, she is beautiful and you look so happy," said Liu.

Pei Ke had to agree her baby was beautiful. He wondered when he would be able to have a child of his own. First, he needed to have a wife. He looked at Liu and the patients in the ward and then back to the woman's baby. Would he be able to support a family?

"I will do an acupuncture treatment on you today, and I want you to come back here tomorrow for another treatment," said Liu. "You will also need to take some Chinese herbs to stimulate your system. I am going to write a prescription for you to take to your local herbalist. The prescription will help you produce more milk. You may feel your breasts becoming more distended, but they should not be painful."

"Thank you. When will I start to have more milk?"

"You should have a little more milk by tomorrow if you follow my advice and take the herbs today and get good nutrition."

"Pei Ke," said Liu. "I want you to hold her baby while I do the acupuncture treatment. You can still watch."

Pei Ke awkwardly took the baby. He wanted to be a doctor not a nurse.

The woman looked at Pei Ke and said, "Doctor, do you have children?"

"No," said Pei Ke. "I am not married."

He was about to tell the woman he was not a doctor, but he decided not to. He was enjoying the trust the patient had put in him. It was exhilarating. The feeling could become addictive.

"Master Liu, where are you going to put the needles? You're not going to put one in my nipple, are you?"

"There is a point on the nipple, but it is not used for acupuncture. It is more of a landmark point we use to determine the location of other points. I need to put two needles in the center of your chest."

"I hope this is not going to hurt," interrupted the woman. Pei Ke could hear the apprehension in her voice.

"No, it is not going to hurt. I do have to see your breasts. Would you feel more comfortable if a nurse was here with us?"

"Yes."

"Pei Ke, find a nurse and ask her to join us."

"What do I do with her baby?"

"Hold on to the child. It isn't going to bite. Now go, and be quick about it."

Five minutes later Pei Ke returned with the baby, but no nurse. The woman was covered up and a nurse was standing next to the bed. The woman was smiling. Liu looked at Pei Ke.

"Where have you been? I have already treated her."

"I couldn't find a nurse."

Liu looked disappointedly at Pei Ke and then looked at the woman.

"How do you feel?"

"Fine. It did not hurt. I do feel a little bit of distension in the center of my chest radiating to each breast. Is that good?"

"Yes, that is what I want. You will be fine. You need to lay here for a few minutes. It is important that you have more treatments. We have started the healing process but need to continue it for you and your baby."

Pei Ke noticed there was a needle in one of her fingers. He wondered why a needle would be put in her finger to treat an inability to produce milk. He was about to ask Liu when it dawned on him why the needle was there. He remembered Liu using this special point to treat this problem.

"Master, may I ask some questions on how you diagnosed this problem?"

"Yes."

"How did you know it was a Qi and blood deficiency?"

"Her answers to my questions and her signs and symptoms are the clues. If she indicated she was depressed, her breasts were sore, she had chest pain along with a pink tongue and her pulses were string taught, then I would have diagnosed it differently. That combination would be more in keeping with Liver Qi stagnation. Of course, I would use some different acupuncture points, and the herbal prescription would be different."

The baby started to cry and Pei Ke had no idea what to do. He looked to the mother for help. To Pei Ke's relief the nurse took the baby.

"Master, while I was gone where did you put the needles?"

Liu explained which points he had used and the logic behind each choice. Again Liu emphasized the importance of getting as much information as possible to correctly diagnose the problem.

"Master, this is the second time we have seen a woman who had had difficulty in nursing. Do many women have this problem?"

"It is common enough that you need to be aware of the symptoms and know how to differentiate between the various ways of treating this problem.

For a woman, it is the culmination of nine months of carrying a new life. It should be a happy and joyous time to have a baby. She needs to develop this close attachment to the baby. Nursing is one way this bond is developed. As you saw, the mother was distraught about not being able to nurse. After she was reassured that her problem could be fixed, her demeanor changed."

"Master, what is more important in treating this problem: the acupuncture or Chinese herbs?"

"Actually, either one can work, but together they will be more effective. She needs to come back for more treatments. I would suspect if we see her again her tongue, and pulses will be different."

"You say that with some hesitancy. Do you think she will not return?"

"We will see," said Liu.

"What other problems could have happened because of a Qi deficiency?"

"We asked her if there were any urination problems, and she indicated no. However, incontinence is a common problem after prolonged childbirth, multiple births, and constant pushing downward during delivery."

"Will the same acupuncture points you used for the lack of breast milk also help with the incontinence?"

"No, even though it is a Qi deficiency, it is affecting a different part of the body and needs to be treated with different points based on the differential diagnosis. Incontinence can be due to more than one imbalance so again, it is the diagnosis of where the imbalance exists that is important in solving the incontinence. Do you understand?"

"Yes, Master."

Pei Ke hesitated a few moments as he thought through the next question he was going to ask.

"What other problems can this woman have?"

"After she has started nursing, she needs to have proper care of her breasts and nipples. Many women like to nurse while they are lying down. There is nothing wrong with this, but there is a tendency for the mother and child to fall asleep. In order to produce more milk, the mother needs to make sure the infant has nursed enough to stimulate the breasts to produce more milk. Secondly, the mother needs to make sure she has the proper hygiene before and after nursing. Not cleaning her nipples after nursing can lead to a buildup of milk on the outside of the nipple and breast causing a slight cracking of the nipple. This can cause the breast to become infected. It is very painful."

*There are so many things to remember*, thought Pei Ke. He was deep in thought when Liu continued.

"This woman had the problem of not having enough breast milk. Some women do not want to nurse their baby for one reason or another; or the time for weaning the child has come. There are other acupuncture points to stop the flow of milk. The mother needs to have acupuncture treatments for a few days to accomplish this. During this process she needs to decrease the amount of nursing and increase the amount of solid foods. The amount of solid foods depends on the age of the infant and when solid food was initially introduced.

Liu and Pei Ke went on to see twenty or thirty patients. At the end of the day, Pei Ke was tired but felt he had learned a tremendous amount in a short period of time. He realized what Liu had told him before. There was no substitute for patient contact.

He knew it would take hundreds and hundreds of patients for him to be anywhere as knowledgeable as Liu.

# CHAPTER FORTY-SIX

Liu and Pei Ke arrived at the hospital early on the next day. As soon as they arrived, they were asked to join in on the patient rounds.

"Master, we have an unusual situation with a woman who is nine months pregnant," said the doctor. "She has just arrived at the clinic in obvious distress. I know you are starting to make rounds, but this warrants our attention; it is a life-threatening situation, and we could use your expertise."

"Yes, we will come immediately."

Liu and Pei Ke walked past numerous women and arrived at a special area of the clinic reserved for delivery. Pei Ke was amazed at the number of women who were in different stages of labor.

*This must be a special area for difficult cases*, thought Pei Ke.

Almost all women delivered their babies at home, which is the prevailing custom. The midwife would stay with the mother during this time and help with the birthing process. Only in time of need would the doctor see the mother, and usually the doctor went to the house as needed. Here it was different; the mother came to the doctor.

*There must be a shortage of doctors or a lot of couples trying to have children,* thought Pei Ke.

He'd never known there was such a thing as a doctor until his mother had been really sick and the doctor came to the house. The doctor prescribed some herbs and never came again. He was sure it was because they were so poor. Luckily, she recovered and everything was all right with her.

When he became a doctor, Pei Ke vowed he would make himself available to all patients, regardless of their status, wealth or the inconvenience to him. Liu took care of anyone and had taught him that this was the responsibility one assumes when one decides to enter this profession.

Pei Ke and Liu arrived at the bedside of an obviously pregnant woman. The doctor introduced both Liu and Pei Ke as doctors. Again Pei Ke felt honored to be in the presence of his teacher. He also once again felt honored but burdened with being referred to as a doctor. He wondered if Liu had ever felt this way when he'd first started.

"How can we help you?" said Liu to the woman.

"I am due to have my baby, but the baby won't come out. I am extremely uncomfortable and in a lot of pain. Help me, please."

Liu turned to the doctor and asked. "When did she arrive?"

"She came in yesterday evening. We suspect the baby is in a breech position, needing special attention. We wanted to wait to see if the situation would correct itself, but it is obvious the baby is not going to turn correctly."

"Is this your first pregnancy?" Liu asked the woman.

"No, it is my third. I didn't have this problem with my other babies. Is there something you can do?"

"Yes, we are going to help you to deliver your baby. I do need to ask you some questions first."

"Yes, ask me anything, but help me."

"When did you realize you were pregnant? I need to know the month and day if possible."

"I became pregnant nine months ago. The baby is due now."

"We need to examine your abdomen. Is that all right?"

"Yes."

"Pei Ke, I want you to go and find a midwife."

Pei Ke turned to search for a midwife and was relieved to see one standing right behind him, waiting. She introduced herself and Liu continued with the questions.

"Were your other two pregnancies normal?"

"Yes."

"Did you deliver them at the right time?"

"Yes."

"Was the labor longer or shorter for the second baby?"

"It was shorter and much easier. I was in labor for only twelve hours for the second one. The first one was over twenty-four hours."

"How long have you have been in labor now?"

"Over twenty-four hours."

"Is the progress of your delivery the same as before?"

"No, this one feels entirely different. I don't think the baby wants to be born."

Liu turned to the midwife.

"How far is she along in the process?"

"She is quite far along now and the baby should be descending along the birth canal by now. I feel the baby may be in a breech position."

"Pei Ke do you understand what is happening to this woman and her baby?"

"No."

"Normally, by the time the baby is to be born, the baby's head would be in a downward position so it can be born. Sometimes, for various reasons, the baby does not turn and therefore can't be born normally. It is a life-threatening situation for both the baby and the mother. There is just so much time we can wait for nature to take its course before we have to do something."

"Help me, please," said the expectant woman. She started to cry.

"Master, if the baby is turned the wrong way, how do you get the baby to turn correctly?"

"There is an acupuncture point the ancients discovered that will help both the mother and the baby. It is located on one of the toes and is used for just such a situation as this.

"Some practitioners of Traditional Chinese Medicine believe this special point should be needled. Others feel moxibustion on the point is more appropriate. I feel each situation is unique and the pulses should dictate which method should be used. In some instances, you can do both: first, needling the point and then heating up the needle with the moxa stick to get enhanced results."

"What should we do in this situation?" asked Pei Ke.

"I need to feel the pulses first."

Liu felt the pulses on the right wrist first followed by the pulses on the left wrist. He paid particular attention to the pulses dealing with the spleen, kidney, and liver energies. These were the main energy pulses dealing with women's problems and would be the ones to help him make a decision. He also paid attention to the pulse on the Urinary Bladder Meridian to see if it was basically excess or deficient.

Next, Liu looked at the woman's tongue to see if there were any unusual colors, markings, or coatings.

"Pei Ke, based on the pulses and the tongue diagnosis, I believe we only need to do acupuncture. I want you to feel the pulses and look at her tongue."

Pei Ke took a few minutes to read the pulses and then looked at her tongue.

"Pei Ke, I want you to go back and do it all over again. You were too quick in your pulse reading. You may have read the pulses wrong."

Pei Ke retook the pulses paying particular attention to the spleen, kidney, and liver pulses. Liu was correct; spending more time with the pulse diagnosis helped him to further differentiate the quality of the pulses.

Liu did the acupuncture treatment while Pei Ke watched intently. After they were finished he reassured the woman everything had been done and it was important for her to be calm. He promised that someone would visit with her shortly.

That day the midwife helped deliver a healthy six pound baby. Liu and Pei Ke heard about it later from one of the doctors.

# CHAPTER FORTY-SEVEN

Master Liu, we have a woman complaining of severe menstrual cramps. She heard about our clinic and has come to see one of the doctors. We are exceptionally busy today. Would you be so kind as to see her? If you need anything just ask the nurse."

"Yes, I will be glad to help her. Where is she?"

"She's over there, next to the window. Do you see her?"

"Is she the one holding her abdomen and crying?"

"Yes."

"Pei Ke, do you remember when we treated Mrs. Wang's daughter-in-law for her menstrual cramps?"

"Yes, Master. Once you put the needles in her pain subsided almost immediately. Treating and alleviating her pain almost instantly was one of the factors reinforcing my belief in your abilities and the effectiveness of Traditional Chinese Medicine."

"Menstrual pain is one of the most common conditions affecting women. We, as men, are lucky not to have to experience it. For some women, it is quite debilitating. Every month they can expect to have their monthly menstrual cycle, and the accompanying pain and discomfort. Often they have to plan their lives around when their period starts. Many women remind themselves when their period is to start by placing little marks or notes on the calendar. Some women are very regular and know to the day when they can expect to have cramping. Other women vary from month to month. There are some women who have very irregular cycles.

"It is a mixed blessing for women. For those who are regular in their cycle, they know when they've missed their period and may be pregnant. For them, it is a time to be joyous. For those who did not plan to get pregnant, a missed period is not good news.

"Women comprise approximately half of the population, so as a doctor it is safe to presume that half the time you will be seeing women. Women do have some unique health care issues that we do not have. This is one reason why I brought you to this clinic: so you can gain some experience treating the diversified health issues of women. There is a double benefit to this clinic. Not only do the doctors here treat women, but they also treat children's problems. So you will get to see some of the issues unique to children.

"Before we see this woman, I want to tell you what we can expect to see. In general, when women have a monthly cycle there is some minor discomfort. The woman's body is going through some significant changes. This minor discomfort can be expected since her body is getting rid of old blood and preparing itself for the next cycle. When the period is really painful, there is an imbalance that needs to be corrected.

"Severe pain during a woman's period in Traditional Chinese Medicine is attributed to a couple of different reasons. It can be either an excess condition or a deficiency condition that causes a disruption of flow of Qi and Blood in the uterus. The underlying question is: what causes the disruption of the flow of Qi and Blood?

"For an excess condition, it can be stagnation of liver Qi or the consuming of too many cold drinks and eating too much cold food just before or during the menstrual period. For a deficiency condition, it may be a basic weakness in the body or from chronic diseases.

"Pei Ke, you will need to be able to differentiate between the excess and the deficiency to be able to correctly treat the patient. As you know by now, excess has one set of symptoms and deficiency has another set of symptoms.

"If it is an excess, then the woman will complain about lower abdominal pain, dark purplish menses and clots, breast distension and tenderness, and a purplish tongue with purple spots. The tongue will have a white sticky coating. When you feel the pulses you would expect to feel a deep, string-taut pulse on the Liver position.

"If it is a deficiency, then the woman will have dull pain at the end of the menses flow that is alleviated with either pressure or warmth applied to the abdomen. During the period, the menses will not be dark. She will have an aversion to cold and her extremities will feel cold. Her complexion will be pale and she may have heart palpitations and complain of dizziness. You can anticipate a thready and weak pulse signifying a deficiency condition.

"Pei Ke, can you remember all that?"

"Yes, I think I can remember all that."

"We need to now go over and see her."

Liu and Pei Ke walked the short distance to the patient. Pei Ke was looking forward to the diagnostic process that Liu was going to do on this patient. He knew exactly what to look for and was sure he could follow exactly what Liu was going to do.

As Liu had made the rounds with the other doctors, he'd remembered the process he'd gone through when he was a beginning student. He did not have the luxury of learning and practicing in a hospital, but he had many teachers. His initial teachers taught him because of his father. When he had first expressed an interest in learning Traditional Chinese Medicine, his father had been against it. He had wanted his son to continue in his footsteps and be part of running the family estate.

Liu had pleaded with his father to let him learn medicine, so finally his father had made arrangements with a local doctor to begin his studies. At first he had been allowed to visit with the doctor once a week. The doctor would give him homework which he did diligently. After a couple of months, the doctor had been so impressed with Liu's ability that he had visited with Liu's father and suggested that his son become a doctor.

Liu's father had reluctantly agreed and had let Liu visit with the doctor three times a week. Liu remembered being enthralled with what the doctor could accomplish with just a few needles and some herbs. The more he saw and experienced, the more he wanted to make Traditional Chinese Medicine his life's profession. The concept of helping others less fortunate than him was very appealing. It was a major reason he devoted his life to understanding the Universal Energy of Taoism.

# CHAPTER FORTY-EIGHT

Pei Ke, I want you to go with Dr. Han for the next three days. He will teach you the intricacies of needling techniques, cupping, and moxibustion. You are going to be very busy with him. Do you still have the amulet?"

"Of course, Master."

"Let me see it."

Pei Ke took the amulet from around his neck and gave it to Liu. Liu put it around his own neck.

"Master, what will you be doing? Will you be here at the hospital or are you going out?"

"Is it important for you to know?"

"Forgive me, Master. It was very rude of me to ask. I will do as you say."

For the next three days, Pei Ke watched and practiced needling techniques. First, Dr. Han made sure Pei Ke knew about the characteristics of the various needles. Then, he watched as Pei Ke handled the needles. To feel the coming of the energy in the needle, the needle had to be held in a certain manner.

As he became more proficient, Pei Ke learned more insertion techniques. Dr. Han placed a few sheets of rice paper on top of a towel for Pei Ke to practice on. Next Pei Ke practiced on an orange and finally Dr. Han gave his approval for Pei Ke to do needling on a live person.

"Pei Ke, I want you to take your own pulses, and tell me what you find."

Pei Ke took his own pulses.

"Dr. Han, I have a deficient liver pulse. This is probably the reason I have a headache."

"Do you have any neck pain?" asked Dr. Han.

"Yes," said Pei Ke. "My neck is stiff and I have a headache on the right side of my head."

"With just the information you have gathered so far, would you use either a gallbladder point or a heart point?"

Without hesitating Pei Ke answered.

"Dr. Han, I would use a gallbladder point. If I had to use only one point, it would be either this one or that one."

Pei Ke pointed to the two points he would choose to solve the headache and stiff neck problem.

"Pei Ke, you have been practicing needling techniques for two days. Do you have any questions? Do you feel confident to treat a patient?"

"Yes, I'm confident I can treat a patient. Is there one for me to treat?"

"Would you like to be treated for your headache and stiff neck first?"

"Yes, please," said Pei Ke.

"Sit down and roll up your right pant leg," said Dr. Han.

*It will be interesting*, thought Pei Ke, *to see how good Dr. Han is with acupuncture.* Pei Ke made a mental note of the area where he had the pain and the degree of discomfort he was experiencing. He had experienced headaches like this before. They weren't too frequent, just a couple times a year. They usually went away after a good night's rest. It would be interesting to see how quickly the headache goes away. Pei Ke smiled as Dr. Han walked across the room to get some sterile needles. As Dr. Han was returning, Pei Ke was looking at his leg.

"Are you ready?" asked Dr. Han.

"Yes," said Pei Ke.

Pei Ke looked down at his right leg, waiting for Dr. Han to insert the needles. A couple of seconds later, when nothing had happened, he looked up to see Dr. Han with a handful of needles staring at him.

"You are the doctor," said Han. "It is now time for you to treat yourself. Since you have no questions and are confident in your needling abilities, there should be no problems."

A cold sweat broke out on Pei Ke's forehead as he realized he was going to put a needle into his own leg. Liu should have warned him ahead of time. He needed time to prepare for the procedure.

"Dr. Han, where do you want me to put the needle?"

"I want you to put it into an acupuncture point. Please."

"Which point?"

"Do you have a headache?"

"Yes."

Pei Ke could see the exasperation on Dr. Han's face as Han pointed to an acupuncture point just below Pei Ke's right knee. Pei Ke took one needle from Dr. Han and, with some hesitancy, inserted the needle into his leg. He immediately felt significant pain.

"The first thing I want you to remember is to do no harm to the patient," Han said. "The acupuncture process should not be painful, yet you are experiencing pain. Do you know why?"

"No, Dr. Han."

"The reason you are experiencing pain is you did not put the needle in the correct location. You are off by just a little. In this case, it is the difference between being painful and not painful. Because your needle is not in the right location you still have the headache. Am I correct?"

"Yes," said Pei Ke.

"Take the needle out and try again."

Pei Ke took the needle out of his leg. Han gave him another needle and Pei Ke, after considerable thought and deliberation, inserted the needle again. To his relief, it did not hurt at all.

"Now you have the right location," said Dr. Han. "Did the headache go away?"

"No," said Pei Ke. "In fact, it is now slightly worse."

"Do you know why?"

Pei Ke looked at the needle and quickly realized the needle was inserted somewhat incorrectly. The location was correct but the insertion direction was not. He made the change to the needle and instantly felt the energy move in his leg. The headache and stiff neck went away.

Dr. Han smiled.

"Think about what you have learned," said Dr. Han.

# CHAPTER FORTY-NINE

On the seventh day at the hospital, Liu and Pei Ke worked late. Pei Ke was exhausted, but it felt good to be of service to those in need. They said goodnight to the staff as they closed the door and walked down the steps to the dimly lit street. The moon was hidden by the overcast skies. Light showing through windows only minimally helped them make their way down the street. This was the first time they had worked so late.

They were no more than a block from the hospital when three men suddenly and with no visible warning attacked from one of the adjoining dark alleys. Even Liu with his ability to sense danger had missed the coming attack.

One man grabbed Pei Ke's sack while another punched him in the chest. As Pei Ke reeled from the blow he also felt the straps of the sack being ripped from his arms. He desperately held on to the sack remembering Liu telling him he must protect the sack and its contents at all costs.

As the sack slipped down his arms, he relaxed and turned into the force of the pull. Pei Ke lunged forward and threw his left arm around the sack. With his right arm he punched the man with all the power he could muster. He felt his fist make contact with the man's nose. Pei Ke immediately followed up with finger jabs to both eyes.

The other man grabbed Pei Ke's wrist and tried to separate Pei Ke from Liu. With one quick motion Pei Ke used one of the Chin Na moves Liu had taught him and was out of the grab. He turned to find Liu calmly watching him fight, his attacker already running away. The two on Pei Ke quickly followed.

"It lacked finesse, but it will do," said Liu. "Your reactions are still too slow. You should have blocked the punch."

"Master, they wanted the sack."

"I know," said Liu. "You did fine in protecting the sack, but you should have blocked the punch as well."

"Do you think they will be back again tonight?"

"No, the fight has been taken out of them for the night."

They continued down the street. Pei Ke was no longer tired. Liu was deep in thought and needed to make plans. Chen Chang had brought the fight to the streets of Beijing.

―――――――――

Chen Chang watched the altercation from a distance. He had hired the three men to get the sack. He should have told them to kill Liu and the boy. He admonished himself for not leading the attack. He would have killed at least Liu when the other three had attacked.

He needed to find out what is in the sack. Maybe it contained some of the Liu family fortune. Whatever it was, Liu and the boy were intent on protecting it.

# CHAPTER FIFTY

It would be another two hours before the early morning sun made its appearance. Liu and Pei Ke walked briskly along one of Beijing's deserted streets.

"Master, where are we going? You seem to be in a hurry."

"We are going to the park. Yesterday, one of the students of my friend—the man we met in the park—brought me a note inviting us to meet with him early this morning."

"Who is he? What does he want? He wasn't very pleasant when we spoke with him before."

"He is Master Wen. He is well known for his Hsing-Yi Chuan. I do not know what he wants. We used to be good friends. We had many good conversations and spent many hours training together. The note sounded conciliatory and genuine so maybe he wants to rekindle our past friendship. If so, I look forward to it. If not, we will hear him out. Almost everyone I knew in Beijing has either passed away or moved on. It would be nice to have some good memories of our stay here."

"Master, is he good in martial arts?"

"He is well versed in more than one martial art and would make a formidable enemy. When we trained together we were evenly matched. Of course, there were some things in which he excelled and some things in which I excelled, but overall we were well matched. Our teacher recognized our abilities, which is one of the reasons he had us train together so much."

As they walked along the streets, the smells of the city changed as they went from one street to another. The faint smell of tofu was replaced by cooking oil and Yue Tao. Pei Ke was getting hungrier by the minute.

They entered the park as they had done before. There was no one in sight and they walked along the same path they'd walked days earlier. It would be an hour or more before the regular crowd of practitioners showed up for their morning training.

Liu was in bright spirits as they rounded the corner at the far end of the park and went to the scheduled meeting area. In the moonlit darkness, Liu and Pei Ke saw the outline of two men in a small clearing. The clearing was surrounded on three sides by dense foliage, giving the spot the feeling of real seclusion.

"I didn't think you would come," said Wen, as they entered the clearing.

Liu smiled sadly.

"I have come out of respect for our past friendship. Once, we were close friends and I would like to see that friendship rekindled. We are both old men now and it would be nice to know that at our age we can call our friendship lasting."

"Our friendship ended on those last days before you mysteriously departed for places unknown."

"I left because I did not want there to be any misunderstanding between me and our teacher. It was a mistake for him to put us in competition against each other in the tournament. We were evenly matched."

"You won by trickery," said Wen.

"It was not trickery," said Liu. "It was a valid martial arts move that you had never seen before. You reacted wrongly and I did what any martial artist would do and used your movement and reaction to your disadvantage. I remember it distinctly. There is no reason why you should hold that against me. You would have done the same."

"Even Teacher was surprised to see such a move," said Wen.

"We all came to Teacher with prior experience. I used what I knew as you did. You made such a big deal before the competition about how you were going to win, that you backed yourself into a corner you could not escape without losing face. I left so that there would be no conflict between you and me and our teacher."

"We will resolve who is best here and now."

"I have no desire to do this," said Liu. "We were friends once and I want us to depart today as friends again."

"We will never be friends again."

With those words, Wen lunged with a half-hearted punch to Liu's face. At the same time, Wen's student made his move against Pei Ke. Liu was ready, but Pei Ke was not.

Wen was waiting for Liu to make a countermove before he unleashed his powerful Bung Chuan punch to Liu's midsection. If the punch were to make contact, as it was intended, the fight would be over. But as Liu blocked the weak first punch, he knew it was not the main attack and he prepared for whatever was to come. With one swift move he coiled around the force of the second punch, deflecting it to his right.

Pei Ke was not as lucky. His attacker stepped in and pushed hard with both hands against Pei Ke's chest, throwing him to the ground. Pei Ke was startled by the movement, but immediately rose and readied himself for the next attack. In the back of his mind, he could hear Liu's teaching. His master's words flooded through his mind as he tried to remember all the things he needed to do to win this encounter. Above all, he realized he had to keep moving to keep his opponent off guard.

Pei Ke took up the ready position of Pa Kua Chang and started to circle to his left as fast as he could. As he circled, he sat into a lower and lower position. This increased his rootedness to the ground and gave him the advantage against any grappling techniques his opponent tried on him.

His swiftness caught his opponent off guard. Wen's student tried to compensate for his bad position, but he shifted too much and Pei Ke had already changed direction. Frustrated, Pei Ke's opponent opened his arms and threw them around Pei Ke in a crushing bear hug.

Liu fared better. After deflecting the second punch, he formed a ball with his right hand over his left and grabbed Wen's right arm. He turned to the right, locking out his opponent's right arm then continued turning while he opened both shoulders. The pain would be instant and Wen's right arm would thereafter be useless.

Liu felt the arm break as he applied the massive torque of his turning waist. It was the turning waist movement that broke Wen's arm and the force and structure of the ball that made this movement so powerful. Liu had watched many Pa Kua Chang practitioners over the years and he often wondered why most of them did not realize that in coiling techniques it was not only the coiling, but also the ball that made Pa Kua Chang so powerful. He was thankful that he had been shown this technique.

Pei Ke felt his body being tightly squeezed and he was about to panic when he remembered what Liu had told him about the value of Hsing-Yi Chuan. There were only five basic moves, Liu had said, but they could handle most street situations. From his low initial position, he brought his hands to the center line of his body and he opened his shoulders, which caused a small space between himself and his opponent.

He'd practiced the Pi Chuan movement of Hsing-Yi Chuan many times and he had dreamt about it, and so this was the move that he used.

The fist was unique to Hsing-Yi Chuan. He placed the second joint of his index finger past the closed fist, and supported it with his thumb. The rigid, protruding, finger would make all the difference when his fist came in contact with flesh.

Pei Ke punched into the hollow space that separated them and his protruding index finger caught his opponent in the sternum. Pei Ke increased the angle of his fist, driving it into the centerline of his opponent's chest. Even though the initial contact area was the sternum, the force of the punch slid along to a specific point on the centerline that influenced the heart.

The movements of Hsing-Yi Chuan are by their very nature linear in direction, but Pei Ke had been taught the value of a rotating surface. From the moment he had made contact with the linear force, he rotated his arms. His right arm rotated one direction and the left arm rotated the other, which was what made the punch so effective.

The pain was so intense that Wen's student immediately released his crushing bear hold and stepped back, giving Pei Ke a chance to continue with the second part of Pi Chuan. He took his right hand and grabbed his opponent's right wrist and pulled him forward. With his left hand, he struck his opponent in the collarbone with the edge of his left hand. The bone split. Liu told him later that the collarbone would never heal correctly.

Someone touched his shoulder from behind, a right hand by the placement of the thumb and fingers. He immediately spun to his right and into the Dragon Palm ready position of Pa Kua Chang. He started to circle behind whoever had touched him when he realized it was Liu.

"Enough," said Liu. "It is I."

They looked at each other than at their opponents. Inwardly, Liu smiled at what he saw. Finally, Pei Ke was coming into his own as a martial artist.

Wen and his student were in obvious pain as they walked away from the altercation. Wen had a broken arm and his student had a broken collarbone. They were both mumbling something, but Liu could not hear what it was.

"Pei Ke you did well."

"Master, I think I broke his collar bone."

"Was the Pi Chuan move difficult for you to execute?"

"No, Master," said Pei Ke. "It was almost effortless."

"Good. That is the way it should be," said Liu. "Let us go."

They began to leave the park and had walked in silence for a few steps before Pei Ke spoke.

"Master, I'm sorry this happened between you and your friend."

"I am sorry as well. It seems that most of my friends and teachers are gone."

"You know the people at the hospital."

Liu turned to look at Pei Ke. He thought about Ming Hong and her son. He wondered what type of man the boy was going to grow up to be. He really needed a father to guide him through the intricacies of life. He was about to say something to Pei Ke when the bushes rustled ahead of them.

Three young men stepped out of the bushes and walked eagerly towards them.

"We watched the whole thing," one of them said. "We're so happy you won. Wen has boasted for many years that he was your teacher's best student. He beats his students unmercifully if they don't do exactly as he tells them and is always saying bad things about the other teachers in the area. No one likes him.

"But we've heard about you from some of the older students. Your reputation is outstanding, not only for your martial arts ability but for your fairness and kindness. We were hoping that you would stay and teach us. Would you please stay?"

Liu was caught off guard by the request. He looked at Pei Ke, then replied.

"I appreciate your invitation, however; I cannot stay now. I must go to resolve some personal matters, but there is a good possibility that I will return to take care of some unfinished business. If I do, then I would be happy to teach you and everyone else that wants to learn. But you must excuse us now."

The young man that was talking to Liu turned to Pei Ke and said. "We watched you defend yourself against one of Wen's better students. Your form and precision were faultless. What secret did Liu teach you that you can share with us?"

Without hesitating Pei Ke said. "Practice and strong legs."

"What else?" shouted one of the men, as Liu and Pei Ke walked away.

Pei Ke looked at Liu and Liu nodded.

Pei Ke turned and shouted. "A rotating surface always works better than a non-rotating surface."

Liu smiled as they neared the gate. The early morning crowd was just beginning to arrive and he was sure that those who had witnessed the fight would tell everyone about it. And Wen would have to explain his injuries.

They walked away from the park. It was time for him to finish his stay at the hospital. There was only one more piece of unfinished business in Beijing and they would be leaving.

# CHAPTER FIFTY-ONE

Master, we have been in Beijing for almost two weeks. We have been to the park twice and the clinic numerous times. We have paid respect at the gravesites of your teachers. Where are we going today? Are we going back to the clinic or are we going to see some of your other friends and teachers?"

"We are going to see an old friend who can help me solve a mystery."

"What is the mystery?"

"My family has had our ancestral land for quite some time. It was the custom in past generations to reward those who were loyal to the ruling emperor by giving them land. The valley and surrounding area was given to our family for service well done. It was recorded with the official seal on a scroll and given to our family. That scroll has been in safe keeping at my brother's house. I took it when we were visiting the graves, and you have been carrying it for the last few days. The assailants we fought last night probably wanted the scroll, which they must have correctly assumed was in the sack."

"Master, I remember you looking at the scroll."

"My old friend may be able to help me find out why Chen Chang thinks he has a claim to the land. My father once mentioned such a possibility, but dismissed it as illegitimate. It is important to put an end to this claim once and for all. I want the land to pass to Hua Yee and the remaining nephews and nieces without dispute."

Liu looked at Pei Ke, and Pei Ke could see a small smile on his face. Pei Ke thought about what Liu had just said. Was there an additional meaning in that statement or was he reading too much into what Liu had just said?

As they walked, Liu reminisced about his childhood in the valley he knew so well, the valley that may now be in danger. It had been an ideal place for someone to grow up. Everything one could want was in the valley. His grandfather had set the foundation and direction for the family. His father had continued the process. His mother had been the one who made everything in the house run smoothly.

His favorite time of year had been autumn. When the weather turned cool and the harvest was over, the family could enjoy the fruits of their labors. He loved the peaches, which were sweet and plentiful. His mother would cut them into small pieces and serve them at the end of a meal. On occasion, she would take the peaches, especially if they were too ripe, and mix the cut pieces with rice and heat it up. The taste was unbelievable. He missed these simple things and, above all, he missed his parents. They were a wonderful influence on his development and he was indebted to them for all they had given to him. If he could only go back and say thank you to them.

He wondered what he would have done if he had married and had a family. *It wasn't the path for him*, he thought. He looked at Pei Ke and saw the similarity between them. A slight tear formed in Liu's eyes as he thought about what might have been. Liu turned and looked at Pei Ke. He was young and had his whole life ahead of him. He looked back briefly on all that he had accomplished—he had no regrets. Liu was brought back to the present by Pei Ke's question.

"Master, do you know where we are going? We seem to be walking aimlessly down the street."

Liu stopped to get his bearings and smiled.

"Yes, I remember the direction. We are not far from where we need to be."

Liu and Pei Ke continued walking for another half an hour until they came to a very ornate building.

"Pei Ke, no one is allowed into the Forbidden City except for the emperor and those who serve him. However, to conduct business it is sometimes necessary to have someone knowledgeable who can answer questions. My old friend Sun Han can help us with the mystery. The last I knew he worked here in one of the official buildings of the emperor."

They opened the door and walked into an open waiting room. A young man sat behind a nondescript desk. As they walked in he rose and looked at them sternly.

"We do not give handouts here. You two are in the wrong place. If you don't leave immediately, I will call the guards and have you arrested for trespassing. This is a government building for government activities only."

"My name is Liu Bin. I am looking for Sun Han. He is a friend of mine."

The man behind the desk looked at Liu and Pei Ke for a moment.

"How do you know Sun Han? He is a respected official in this office. It seems very unlikely that you know him. Clearly you heard his name from someone else. What is your business here?"

"Sun Han is an old friend of mine going back many years. If you mention my name, he will see me."

"Wait here," said the receptionist.

The man disappeared behind a door. Moments later, a different man entered, looked at Liu and Pei Ke, and disappeared. Finally, Sun Han opened the door, looked at Liu, and then smiled.

"Liu Bin, it is a surprise to see you. Come into my office."

Liu and Pei Ke walked into the office. It was as nondescript as the outer waiting area. Both rooms were in sharp contrast to the ornate appearance of the building's exterior.

There was a large desk cluttered with papers and scrolls. It was obvious Sun Han was busy with some type of government work. Numerous book shelves lined two of the walls. Two chairs sat in front of the desk and two more were along one wall. The office was nothing like what Pei Ke would anticipate for a government official's office.

"Please have a seat. Who is this with you?"

Liu introduced Pei Ke who bowed low. Sun Han gave a slight bow in return. Liu motioned for Pei Ke to take a seat as Liu and Sun Han sat down. Liu explained to Sun Han what had happened and why he was visiting with him.

"Pei Ke," Sun Han said, turning to the younger man. "Your teacher and I go back a long way. We trained together in martial arts. He saved my life once and for this I am grateful. You have apprenticed yourself to an outstanding martial artist and teacher." He turned to Liu.

"It is interesting you have come today. A couple of days ago, there was a similar inquiry from a man named Chen Chang. He wanted me to authenticate the scroll he had concerning property west of here in the mountains. I didn't know the land in question belonged to your family.

"I explained to him that the scroll he had, which gave his grandfather specific land, had the seal of a warlord who had lived in the area many years ago. As you know, it was customary for warlords to promise land to individuals who joined them. Of course, the land was not given to just anyone, but to people of power and influence who could bring others to the ranks of the warlords."

As Liu listened to what was being told him, he mentally chastised himself for not coming earlier. It might have saved a lot of time and hardship.

"As different warlords came and went," said Sun Han, "many people received promises of land. As long as a warlord was in power, the landowner would have the protection of the warlord. If the warlord changed, there was no guarantee that the title to the property would be the same.

"In remote areas, like the land your ancestors claim, it was difficult for the emperor to maintain a presence and therefore settle disputes over land. If you have a claim on the land, then I need to see if the document you have, which I presume is a scroll, is legitimate. A legitimate document would have the official wording and official seal of the emperor. Such a document would have first claim over the land. Do you have such a document?"

"Are there records here in Beijing concerning land in the west?" asked Liu.

"Unfortunately, our records are not complete. We need to see the original document signed by the emperor so we can compare the seal on the document with the official seal. If you do not have the document, then it is one person's word against another as to who owns the land."

Liu opened the sack Pei Ke was carrying and took out the scroll and gave it to Sun Han. Sun Han carefully untied the knot and unrolled the scroll, spreading it out on his desk. From inside his shirt, he took out a piece of paper and unfolded it. By the creases on the paper Pei Ke could tell it had been folded in many different directions. On the creased paper was the official seal of the emperor.

Sun Han read the scroll a couple of times and asked Liu a few questions about the land and its boundaries as he knew them to be. Liu remembered his father telling him certain landmarks that delineated the valley and surrounding mountains.

Sun Han looked at the official seal of the emperor. He took the creased piece of paper and folded the paper along one of the creases. The crease was along one side of the seal. He then put the paper on the scroll so that the edge of the seal on the paper lined up with the edge of the seal on the scroll.

When a seal was made, it had very distinctive characteristics. It would be difficult for anyone to make a seal exactly like another seal. There would almost always be some kind of difference or imperfection. It was like handwriting. Someone could try to imitate another's handwriting, but an expert could almost always tell a forgery.

Sun Han turned the paper in many different directions, always matching one side of the paper with its corresponding side on the scroll. Sun Han even noted the width of the lines both on the outside of the seal and the characters on the inside of the seal. He spent about ten minutes turning and folding the paper in every conceivable direction. Each time he matched one surface with another. He looked for oddities on the paper and matched them with corresponding oddities on the scroll. When he was satisfied with the examination, he looked up at Liu.

"The scroll is authentic, and it looks like your ancestors had received rightful ownership to the land. However, I need to caution you about your land. First of all, the emperor has claim to all land. He only allows you to use the land at his convenience.

"Second, does the land pass to you in a natural succession? The natural succession for you would be a document showing that the person named on this document passed the land to someone else. The person who received the land then needs to pass it on to someone else. Maybe your father or brother sold the land to someone else, and you were not informed. Usually, there is a document in safe keeping outlining the succession.

"Third, there are very inadequate records of what land belongs to whom. It is documents like this that we rely on for ownership. If you were to lose this document there would be no way for us to verify that the emperor gave the land to your ancestors.

"Fourth, land needs to have very specific boundaries. This document only gives generalities to the location of the land. Questions could come up as to exact boundaries. Exact boundaries would be from a commonly recognizable location to another commonly recognizable location. Do you have other documents or scrolls delineating the specifics of the land?"

Liu remembered going with his father when he was very young. His father took him to a high point in the mountains and showed him a boulder that had carvings on it. He was young and didn't pay too much attention. He wished now that he had paid more attention. He also remembered his father instructing him about the temple and Kuan Yin hiding place. He was sure there was more to the story about the land. It had to be back at the temple.

"Is there anything else I need to know about this document or about claims to the ancestral land? I now know that I should have come here as soon as we arrived in Beijing."

"When Chen Chang was here, his document described the land as mountainous with a beautiful valley. There was no name to the valley, but there was a very brief description of a mountain pass as a landmark with the land in question lying to the east and west of the mountain pass. Of course, that could describe hundreds of places. I am going to make a written note about what has happened. If Chen Chang shows up again I will handle the situation for you. Right now there is nothing I can do.

"Just be careful about your visit here to Beijing. Times have changed since you were last here. Sometimes the streets are not safe. The population has soared as peasants have flocked to the city in search of work."

Liu nodded his understanding of the situation.

"Where are you staying?" asked Sun Han.

"We are staying with friends," answered Liu. "When I was living here, we had many mutual friends. Do you keep in contact with them?"

"Almost everyone we knew has either passed on or left the area. I know your friend is still here. He has taken over many of our teacher's students."

"I saw him in the park," said Liu.

"Have you inquired about your acupuncture teachers?"

"Yes, it seems they have passed on also. It is a shame they are gone. I learned so much from them. It would be nice to ask them questions and to share with them my own experiences."

"Old friend, can I give you some advice?"

"Of course," said Liu.

"There is nothing more I can do for you here. You need to resolve the conflict with the land. Is Chen Chang reasonable enough that you can talk with him and show him you are the rightful owner of the lands?"

"I do not think so. Too much has happened and he has committed too much to see clearly. As long as there is some doubt about the ownership then he is going to pursue it to the end."

"When he was here, I asked him where he was staying. He mentioned he was staying in the Hu Tong areas west of the West Gate."

Pei Ke immediately recognized the area. They were staying in the same area. Pei Ke looked at Liu, but there wasn't a change in his expression or any indication that he knew the area. Pei Ke hoped he himself had not given away any indication he knew the area.

"Did he indicate where or with whom he was staying," asked Liu.

"He mentioned someone but I didn't pay much attention to it."

"Would there be any reason for Chen Chang to come back to see you?" asked Liu.

"Probably not," said Sun. "I gave him as much information as I had. There was nothing more for me to give him and I indicated as much. I did tell him he needed to solidify his claim. One way would be for him to show the exact boundaries of the land and any buildings. If he could somehow document this with the local authorities, he would have a stronger claim to the land. It would also depend on what Chen Chang would do for the emperor.

"Of course I didn't know at the time that this was your land. I suggested he go back to the area and resolve the details. If there were no other individual or documented claims to the land, maybe the emperor would consider letting him have the land. It would depend on the status of the last warlord who controlled the area.

"He did ask me if there were any known claims or decrees by the emperor on the land. I explained to him the same thing I explained to you about the lack of detailed records. I also explained that any living descendants might have a claim to the land if the local magistrate could somehow document their continued use of the land from one generation to another. If there were no living claimants it would help solidify his cause."

Pei Ke suddenly realized that Hua Yee and the younger children were in imminent peril. If Chen Chang could eliminate Hua Yee and the children along with Liu, he could lay claim to the land. Pei Ke touched the amulet hanging around his neck. He wondered if Chen Chang knew of its existence. If he did, then he would want everyone associated with the four pieces killed. That included anyone who was wearing the amulet. A shudder went down his spine. Did Liu realize the danger his niece was in at the moment? If Chen Chang got there first who knew what he would do?

"Sun, I need a favor from you."

"I am indebted to you for saving my life. Just name it and if it is feasible, I will do it."

"We need fast sturdy horses, but I have no way to pay for them."

As soon as he asked his question, he felt a shift in the Universal Energy. Pei Ke felt the shift as well, though he had never felt such a feeling. It was a feeling of foreboding. He looked at Liu and knew Liu had felt the same thing. They needed to go and go soon.

As they left Sun, eyes followed them as they turned left towards the outskirts of Beijing. Pei Ke turned as he felt something or someone staring at him. Liu had seen and felt the same thing, but said nothing to Pei Ke. They had to walk fast to get to the corral where the horses were kept.

———————

Hua Yee woke up in the middle of the night. She had never had a nightmare this bad. In her dream someone was chasing her and she couldn't get away. The person chasing her knew who she was, but she did not know him. He had a sword and was trying to back her into a corner in a deserted alley.

At the last minute, Pei Ke appeared and swooped her off her feet and carried her to safety. Maybe the dream is an omen of something sinister about to happen. Even though the dream was frightening, she knew Pei Ke was coming back. Or was he?

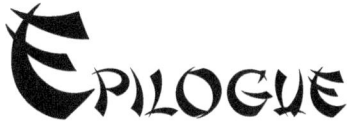

# EPILOGUE

C hen Chang and his men had a substantial lead over Liu and Pei Ke, and they were on horseback. Liu desperately needed to get some horses and to get them fast so he could get back home. Hua Yee, the younger children, and Mr. Wu were in imminent danger and he was over two hundred miles away. If Chen got there first he shuddered to think of what would happen to them. The only solution was for Liu and Pei Ke to travel by horseback.

It had been many years since he last rode a horse. He didn't know if Pei Ke had ever ridden before. If not, he was going to soon learn.

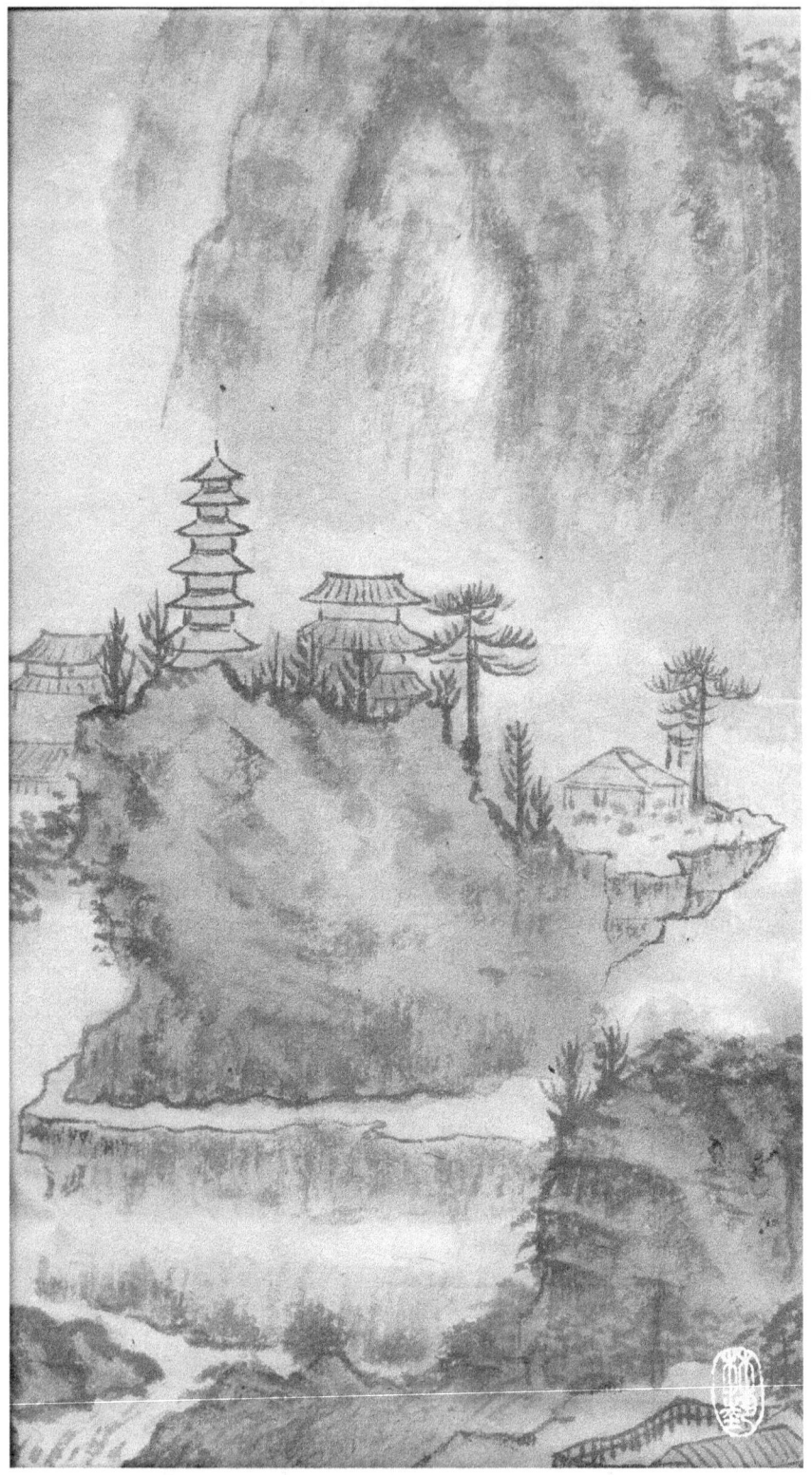